EDDIES
OF THE
KERN

Looking Back

BY TIMOTHY LEMUCCHI

Acknowledgments

*T*he motivation to write this book comes largely from my dear sister Tonia Valpredo who would often admonish me: "Why don't you write a book about all those crazy things you do so I don't have to continually explain to my friends where you are, what crazy thing you are up to now and try to give them the details of your latest escapade. If you write a book," she would say, " I can just tell my friends, 'read the book!'." Well Tonia, here it is!

I also want to thank my adventurous wife, Margaret, my life travel companion, and my daughter, Lisa, who were companions with me on many Alaska adventures, and particularly Margaret, a retired English teacher, for her timeless work editing and proofreading.

Many thanks again to the people who helped me put this book together: my graphic designer Ana Reyna who did beautiful work on the cover design layout and color photography and Candi Asuncion, my transcriptionist.

Sincere thanks also to my adventurous companions many of whom are named in the stories herein who accompanied me on these adventures, provided support and companionship which allowed me to visit and experience some of the most spectacular and scenic environments on this planet.

Timothy Lemucchi
Fall 2020

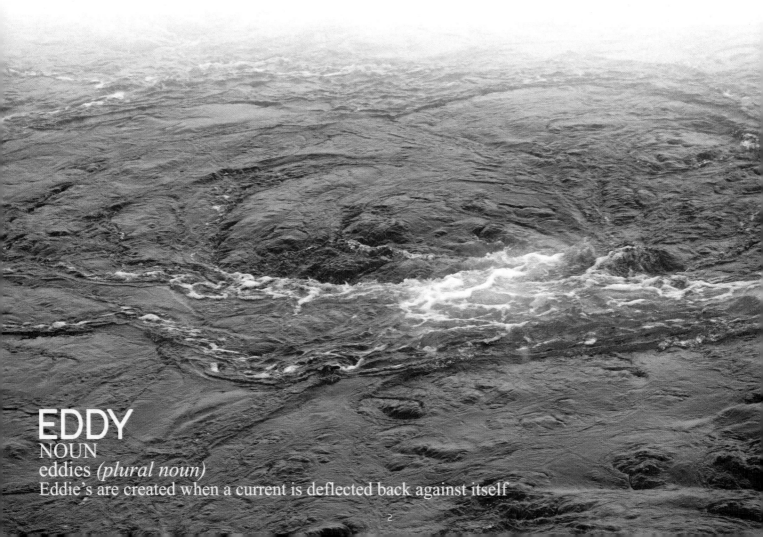

EDDY
NOUN
eddies *(plural noun)*
Eddie's are created when a current is deflected back against itself

The Chapters
EDDIES OF THE KERN

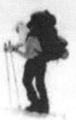

LIFE ON THE RIVER

Bakersfield, California, my hometown where I was born and raised, is situated in the southern end of the San Joaquin Valley - California's great valley - in a hot, dry, aired, semi desert-like environment. The south end of the valley is in a partial rain shadow boarded on the west by the coastal mountain range and on the east and south by the Sierra Nevada Mountains and the Tehachapi Mountains. This end of the valley ekes out less than six inches of rain a year but even so Kern County, the political jurisdiction that occupies the south end of the valley is an agricultural phenomenon producing more than 250 different varieties of crops and is one of the most agriculturally productive areas in the United States, an amazing achievement with such little rain fall. This is accomplished by irrigation with water from outside the southern end of the valley: the natural flow of the Kern River which drains the central and southern Sierra Mountains; the California Aqueduct which transports water throughout the state from the Yuba River in northern California; the Kern Friant Canal which brings water to Kern County from the San Joaquin River which drains the central Sierra Nevada Mountains; and the Central Valley Aquifers which are continuously pumped to make up for short falls in the agricultural water needs.

I have been enthralled and captivated by the history, the beauty and the majesty of the Kern River, the natural water source for our end of the San Joaquin Valley, for over seventy years. My love affair with this river began as a youth in the early 1940s when my father and grandfather would take me as a child on tree mushroom hunts along the Kern River's flood plane below the China Grade Bluffs on the north edge of the city of Bakersfield. We would have to trudge through the heavy riparian growth along the south banks of the river to break into the main river body flowing strong and wide through its channel. I used to wonder where all this water came from and how did it get here. My dad told me that the water came from the High Sierra Mountains and flowed some-two hundred miles before it arrived in Bakersfield. For a young boy this was quite puzzling. I used to wonder how this happened and as I grew older I would continue to explore the banks of the river and be amazed at the volume of water that I would encounter. I would ride my bike to the area below Columbus Street and Union Avenue and explore alone or with my friends this mystical body of water "that came from the High Sierras."

What are the High Sierras, I wondered?

I remember vividly in the 1950s standing on the bluffs across from Bakersfield College and seeing the results of an excessive winter runoff of rain and snow melt that had flooded the entire area below the bluffs as far as one could see, the water even penetrating into downtown Bakersfield, with water on Chester Avenue, the main street of town. The Lake Isabella Dam was not completed until 1966. Before the Dam's completion the Bakersfield town area was often flooded in the Spring. The Chester Avenue Bridge was saved only when county crews put cranes on the bridge and removed driftwood and debris as it accumulated against the east side bridge piers. The water level almost reached the 99 freeway but the levy system prevented flood waters from doing a lot of damage to downtown Bakersfield. The year 1966 proved how important Lake Isabella Dam was to Bakersfield. The crest of the great 1966 flood above Isabella Lake at Kernville was more than 100,000 cubic feet per second - the highest water ever recorded on the river. Isabella Lake completely filled and water floated over the spillway of the dam. If the dam had not been completed engineers calculated all of Bakersfield would have been swept away causing billions in damages.

In my late 60s I fulfilled a lifelong dream and ambition and purchased a two and a half acre parcel on the north bank of the river and moved into my river house with my family, dogs and cat. My river home has over 360 feet of river front and comes with an assortment of fauna and flora so the living there is like being in the midst of a game preserve.

Since I became a river dweller I immersed myself in the daily published statistical information available to measure the daily current and flow of the river from the Kern Canyon. Watching these numbers I have seen the flow as high as 5,500 cubic feet a second and as low as 100 cubic feet a second. CFS or cubic feet per second stands for the amount of cubic feet of water that passes a measuring point in one second. It is an accepted measure of gaging a river's flow. The CFS is largely determined by the amount of rain, snow and spring snow melt in the central and southern Sierra Nevada Mountains the source of the Kern River's water.

Since becoming a river dweller one of my favorite pastimes is to sit on the lower terrace at my house a few feet above the river's surface and watch the mesmerizing ebb and flow of the river currents. It can change from season to season and with the hour of the day. The pleasure of this experience can be enhanced by a hot cup of coffee in the mornings or a glass of Pinot Noir in the late afternoon. One current feature that is always almost present in the river's flow is the Eddies.

Eddies are created when a current is deflected back against itself like a metaphoric look back. As I watch the ebbs and flows of the river and the eddie's I thought that this was an excellent way to describe my accumulated stories herein, a metaphoric "look back," hence "Eddies on the Kern."

The stories related herein are a metaphoric look back at some of the experiences and adventures that I have participated in that others might find interesting. On many of the adventures I write about I kept a daily journal so that the descriptions are fairly accurate as to the events, dates, times and places. If I did not keep a daily journal I always took photographs so that much of a journey and the sequence of events could be recreated from the photo record. Sit back, relax and enjoy being carried along by the Eddies of the Kern.

Timothy Lemucchi
Fall 2020

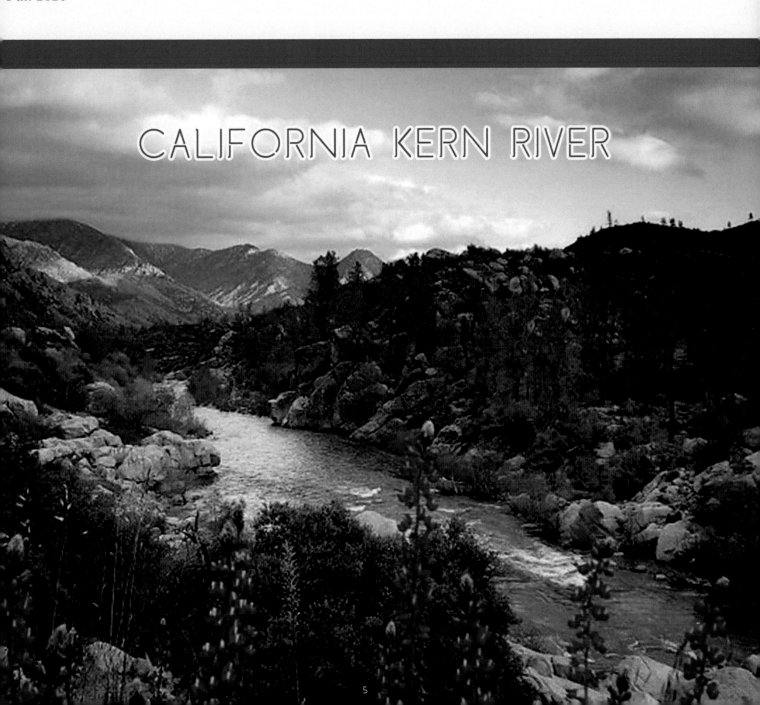

CALIFORNIA KERN RIVER

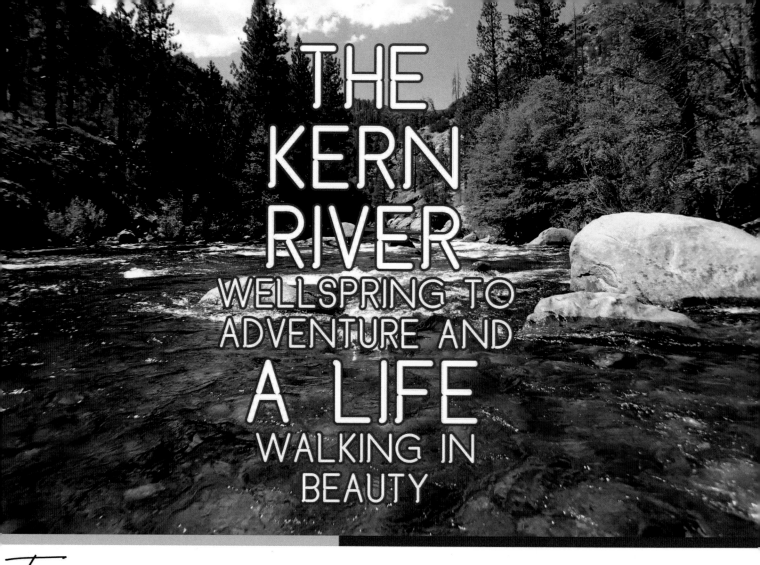

THE KERN RIVER
WELLSPRING TO ADVENTURE AND
A LIFE
WALKING IN BEAUTY

The great thing about the Kern River is that it not only flows through the town where I was born and raised and just a few blocks from my family home as a youth but for the last twenty years as a river dweller the river flows through my backyard. For me the Kern River has become a living entity that I spend time with daily as if it has become a part of the family. I write about the river because in looking back the river created an environment that nurtured a craving for adventure. The river encouraged my urges to see what was beyond the next bend and what was over the next hill and what was at the end of the trail less traveled. As a youth I would ride my bike down dirt roads to the river, wander though the hobo trails to the river and marvel at the amount of water flowing down the river channel and wonder about the Sierra Nevadas the place where my father told me all this water came from. Some studies have indicated that the urge to explore and adventure rises in us innately perhaps within our genome. There is a mutation that pops up frequently in such studies, a variant of a gene called DRD 4 which helps control dopamine, a chemical brain messenger important in learning and reward. Human studies have found that this gene makes people more likely to take risks; explore new places, ideas and generally embrace movement, change and adventure. Evidence to me that I was born with this gene arises from the fact that I was born into an early adventurous California pioneer family. In 1843 my great great grandfather James Williams, then age twenty-nine, and his three brothers - John, age twenty-seven; Isaac, age twenty-one; and Squire, age nineteen - rode their horses some 2,000 miles from Cape Girardeau, Missouri on the Mississippi River across the North American continent to Sutter's Fort on the Sacramento River in Mexican, California. James Williams was my mother, Leah Williams, great grandfather. Since I first learned of the Williams brothers' journey when I was old enough to understand what adults were saying in the early 1940s I had always been fascinated by why the Williams brothers decided to leave their father's 640 acre land grant farm where their family had lived since the 1700s and undertake a 2000 mile journey across North America where they endured incredible hardships, navigated through unmapped country, were chased by Indians who tried to kill them, had their horses stolen and nearly starved to death.

There was also my great great great grandmother, Elizabeth Betsy Patterson, who added adventurism to my gene pool. In the spring of 1844 Betsy Patterson, faced a monumental decision. Her husband Andrew had recently died from the malaria epidemic that had swept through the Missouri-Mississippi River frontier region. Betsy was only thirty-four years of age and had five minor children ages six through fourteen. The prospects for Betsy, a widow, in Jackson County, Missouri in 1844 were at best bleak.

Betsy's father, Isaac Hitchcock - also my great grandfather, then age sixty-four, had been to California in 1833 with Joseph Walker and the Bonneville Expedition and had been with Joe Walker when Walker was the first none-Native American to visit Yosemite in 1834.

Betsy had heard from her father, Isaac, and Joseph Walker and their families, all residents of Jackson County, Missouri, about the wonders of the pacific west and the Republic of Mexico.

Betsy announced her decision to go to California. Undoubtedly her family and friends thought she had lost her mind. Isaac, her father, with a background in mountaineering, fur trading and trapping on a previous trip to California in 1833 was not about to let his daughter and five young grandchildren travel 2,000 miles to California alone. Isaac Hitchcock knew the dangers, distance, hostile Indians, difficulty finding food and water and the hardships that would be encountered. Hitchcock at age sixty-four decided to accompany his family.

Isaac, Betsy and the five children, all minors, joined the Steven Townsand-Murphy Party in 1844 led by Elisha Stevens and left on their 2000 mile journey by covered wagon on May 30, 1844 arriving in California in the winter of 1844. I write about Betsy's adventures in my book The Williams Brothers. Since no one in my family ever asked my ancestors the Williams brothers, Betsy Patterson, or her father Isaac Hitchcock why they took up and made this dangerous trip to California I have had to look for my own answers. After much reading and research into early Western American literature I have found a few answers.

The one I like the best is found in Bernard DeVoto's book Mark Twain's America: ... "an April restlessness, a stirring in the blood, a wind beyond the oaks opening spoke of the prairies, the great desert, and the western sea. The common man fled westward. The thirsty lands swallowed him insatiably."

As DeVoto explains the men and women who went west before 1845 were motivated to see the prairies, the great desert, the Rocky Mountains and the western sea and they had the freedom to go and look.

For me it has always been this same motivation to go and look. I have often experienced "that April restlessness, that stirring in the blood, the wind beyond the oaks opening." My yearnings to go and look took me to many of the places I describe in this book. My early yearnings as a youth were satisfied by my explorations of the Kern River and its tributaries. As I grew older some of my questions about the river, the water and where it came from were partially answered when my cousin Clyde "Cookie" Barbeau, five years older would include me on backpacking fishing trips to some of the tributaries of the Kern: Rush Creek, Bull Run, Peppermint Creek, Erskine Creek, Salmon Creek and others. These ventures were as a preteen and teenager. I learned to live outdoors, cook over an open fire, sleep on the ground and adapt to all sorts of weather. I learned ealy the mountaineering skills that would last me a lifetime. At the age of fourteen my cousin's father, Clyde Barbeau, Sr., and Cookie took me on my first horse packing trip into the high Sierras. We packed out of Mineral King and rode horses over Farewell Gap at 10,500 feet then through the high Sierra country over Coyote Pass at approximately 11,000 feet down the east side of the Kern River Canyon. A few miles below Coyote Pass we camped on Coyote Creek at a camp constructed by a Bakersfield man by the name of Krites. We camped there four days but each day fished either Coyote Creek, Coyote Lakes or took a half day horse ride cross country without trail into the hidden Krites Lake up the canyon from the campsite. Mr. Krites had planted the lake with rainbow trout in the 1930s. Hardly anyone had fished the unknown lake and when we arrived the fishing was fantastic - a fish on almost every cast. Only Mr. Krites and his friends fished the lake before us. The rainbow trout had grown to good size, and we caught many healthy fat fish - 16 to 20 inches in length. We would catch and release most of the fish as uncle Clyde said to let them continue to grow bigger for our next trip. Uncle Clyde had had gotten the directions on how to get to Krites Lake from Mr. Angus

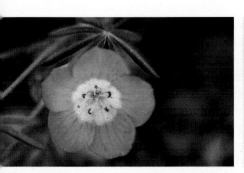
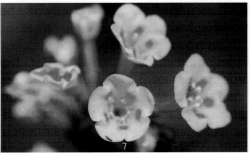
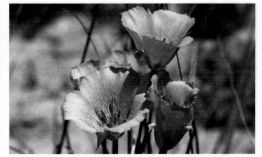

Krites who was a friend. We took some of the freshly caught fish back to Coyote Camp and had delicious fresh trout for dinner and breakfast. The fishing in Coyote Creek was also excellent although the fish were much smaller. Uncle Clyde taught me how to let my bait float down behind the overhanging creek banks and under the rocks where the trout were lurking and then to flip the end of my pole slightly when I felt a tug on the line to set the hook. The fishing lessons learned on Coyote Creek remain with me to this day.

After the trip to Krites Lake I was hooked on adventure, fishing and the high Sierra Nevadas.

After my initial trip with uncle Clyde and cousin Cookie in 1949 I returned to Krites Lake a few more times with my backpacking buddies and once on a horse packing trip with my fraternity brothers from Stanford, Jim McArthur, Bill Juvonen, Bill Tunney and my friend Bobby Carberry and had some fantastic fishing and great wilderness experiences. The focus of my attention for my mountain and wilderness experiences as a young man continued to be with the Kern River and the high Sierras for many years.

In my early forays into the "High Sierras" I usually went with my fishing buddies Fred Perry, Bob Carberry and Rusty Loman. Our choice of beast of burden in those days was usually a donkey as it was the cheapest animal to rent and could carry about 80 pounds including its own food. An accompanying backpacker could carry 50 pounds so two or three travelers could carry very adequate supplies for an extended trip. Horses and pack mules could carry enormous loads (90 lbs.) but were very expensive. It was not until I started practicing law and had the income to support such trips that I could afford the luxury of a horse and mule. Later on when I was able to take such trips the living was grand with good food and supplies that pack animals could transport into the high Sierras. I did visit a great deal of the eastern Sierra high country by pack train, packing out of Reds Meadow Pack Station for several trips and out of Rock Creek Pack Station for several trips and the west side of the Sierras out of Mineral King numerous times.

My first introduction into the incomparable majesty of the eastern high Sierra mountains was in 1948 and 1949 with James Maloney, the Catholic parish priest at St. Joseph's Church. Father Maloney was an outdoor enthusiast and developed a love of the eastern Sierra Nevada from his friend and co-priest John J. Crowley who was the parish priest in Bishop, California in the 1940s. Crowley was well known in the Owens Valley and the eastern Sierras as a priest and a celebrity who worked tirelessly to develop tourism in the Owens Valley after Los Angeles took most of the area water with the Los Angeles Aqueduct to build houses in Los Angeles. Father Crowley's parish stretched from Bishop in the north to Death Valley in the south, a huge expansive territory. Father Crowley inspired Father Maloney's attachment to the beauty of the eastern Sierras. Lake Crowley was named to honor Father Crowley's work for the eastern Sierras.

St. Jude's Church was the Catholic church in Isabella in the 1940s and 50s and was part of Crowley's parish. Father Crowley depended on Bakersfield priests to say mass and provide service to the area parishoners. Father Maloney volunteered to conduct the 6:00 a.m. mass at St. Judes in Isabella, the town that now sits at the bottom of Lake Isabella after the construction of the Lake Isabella Dam by the U.S. Corps of Army Engineers in 1966.

To conduct mass Father Maloney needed alter boys and I and my classmates at St. Joseph Grammar School - John Renfree, Joseph Rostain and David Moffat - volunteered to go with Father Maloney to St. Judes for the 6:00 a.m. mass. The treat that would follow mass would be a trip to the eastern high Sierras. We would all leave Bakersfield at 4:00 a.m. on Sunday, drive on the long winding road up the Kern Canyon to Isabella in time to put our alter boy vestments over our Levis and hiking boots and aid Father Maloney in conducting early mass for the Isabella parishoners. Immediately after mass we would take off the alter boy vestments, load into Father Maloney's 1947 Chevrolet with our tents, sleeping bags and food for the trip to Bishop. At Bishop we would turn left into the Bishop Creek Canyon visiting Lake Sabrina, South Lake or North Lake and the multitude of trail heads, streams and lakes in the Bishop Creek Canyon. We would park the car and take off hiking into the area that Father Maloney had researched and reconnoitered sometimes with the advice of Father Crowley. Father Maloney in those days was in his late 40s or early

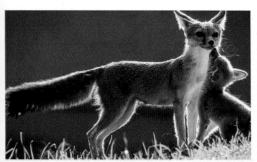
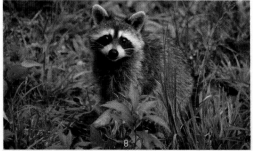
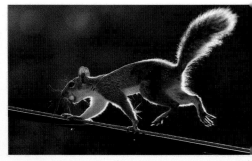

50s and in superb physical condition and would lead our hikes at an accelerated pace. I marvel today how he could negotiate a rock slide bouncing from rock to rock like a ballerina without ever missing a step. We would eat simple food usually prepared by Father Maloney's aides in the church rectory and sleep in single-person pup tents in our sleeping bags. I took several trips with Father Maloney to the eastern Sierras. They were usually two to three days and would cover extensive territory.

I took my first climb of five in all to the top of Mt. Whitney in 1948 with Father Maloney, John Renfree, Joseph Rostain and David Moffat. The first day we climbed to Consultation Lake at 11,000 feet and spent a cold night in our pup tents. The next morning we completed the climb to the summit at 14,500 feet with many "atta boys". On the way back down we glissaded 1,000 feet down a snow filled chute on our rear ends. We saved many tedious switch-backs but in retrospect it was an unsafe procedure but was a blast. We returned to Bishop all too exhausted to drive back to Bakersfield and spent the night in Bishop at the Catholic church sleeping on the floor in our sleeping bags.

On one of the trips after St. Jude's mass we hiked in the mountains and on the way back Father Maloney asked us if anyone had ever been to Death Valley. No one had and he said, "Would you like to see it?" Our answer was, "Of course we would." So off we went to Death Valley adding 200 miles to our trip and arriving there at midnight where the temperature was 120 degrees. It was a long night back to Bakersfield and Father Maloney was so tired that he had us thirteen and fourteen year olds driving his car with Father sleeping in the back seat. We never told our parents who drove.

After climbing Mt. Whitney I heard from my cousin Clyde "Cookie" Barbeau about the incredible fishing at a high mountain lake just north of Mt. Whitney called Wallace Lakes. He told about a way to get into Wallace Lakes by going directly up into and over the Sierra Crest without trail. That fascinated me and I wanted to see if that was possible. Fred Perry and I hiked from the Whitney portal trail head for Mt. Whitney to Inyo Creek Canyon and climbed up the steep canyon without a trail to Boy Scout Lake, then

maneuvered around rock slides eventually coming over the top of the Sierra Crest at Lake Tulainyo, the highest named lake in the continental United States at 12, 818 feet. The lake is quite large over ten acres and usually has some snow all year around the lake. On each of the trips that I made I did try fishing Tulainyo Lake because of old packer tales that there were large fish in the lake. However, I never got any type of a rise or reaction from the lures that I would throw out into the crystal clear waters of the lake. The lake itself is strikingly beautiful with turquoise colored waters. The granite boulders and cliffs in the background of the turquoise water makes it quite a sight. It took some time to work my way down to Wallace Lakes, but the effort was worth it as the fishing in Wallace Lakes in the early 1950s was beyond belief. The lake was full of 20 inch plus beautifully colored fat rainbow trout.

The Kern River is approximately 180 miles long beginning at Lake South America which lies in a high level cirque at 11,000 feet in the Sierra Nevada Mountains. A cirque is an amphitheater-like valley formed by glacier erosion and it is open on the downhill side while the cupped uphill section is generally steep. Lake South America is in a particularly rugged region of the Sierra Nevada Mountains of California just south of Mt. Whitney which at 14,500 feet is the highest peak in the continental United States. My relationship with the Kern River and my curiosity as to where it started and where it goes has over a lifetime taken me over the entire course of the river even to its source at Lake South America both in the summer and in the winter. In the summer I have hiked over Shepherd's Pass, one of the few trailed passes over the eastern escarpment of the Sierras at 12,000 feet and cross-countried off trail into the Lake South America Basin where I camped and fished in its waters. I have also hiked into Lake South America from the western side of the Sierras on the High Sierra Trail which leads into Junction Meadows and where one can follow the dwindling Kern River up into the Lake South America Basin. One memorable horse packing trip in the 1980s with my friends Bill Juvonen and Bobby Carberry we took horses over Franklin Pass North along the river into the upper Kern Canyon, rode north along the Kern Canyon Trail into Junction Meadow where I left the horses at Kern Hot Springs, a natural hot springs near the river and hiked into the Lake South America Basin

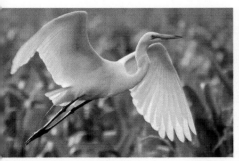

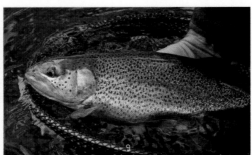

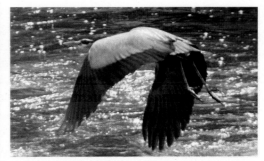

to fish and explore.

In the winter of 1990 I took a ski mountaineering trip into Lake South America as an adjunct to a trans-Sierra crest three week ski tour which I write about herein. We started at Bishop Pass, skied south on the Sierra crest over the highest passes in the Sierras and eventually came to Shepherd's Pass. I skied and climbed over Shepherd's Pass at 12,000 feet covered with snow and ice and snow camped on Diamond Mesa on the plateau above Shepherd's Pass. I was with other skiers but took off on my own and ski traversed back into the Lake South America Basin where there was at least 20 feet of snow on the ground and the lake was frozen over just to experience the isolated winter wonder of the high Sierras and see all that snow and ice in the Lake South America cirque before it thawed and started its long journey down the canyon into the arid flats of the San Joaquin Valley.

I have backpacked, horse-packed and donkey-packed all through the magnificent glacier carved upper Kern Canyon wilderness where I have accessed the Golden Trout Wilderness and caught and released the beautiful golden trout that inhabit Golden Trout Creek. I have also accessed the river over Franklin Pass at 12,000 feet down Rattlesnake Canyon to the river and camped and fished both north and south on the river at Funston Meadows and at the big and little Kern lakes. I have hiked into the river with donkeys over Colby Pass on the High Sierra Trail and into the Kern Kaweah camping at Junction Meadow. I have backpacked over Black Rock Pass down through the Chagoopa Plateau region and into the river.

I have backpacked into the river over Black Rock Pass with donkeys, accessed the river over the Kaweah gap to Hamilton Lakes and the Nine Lakes Basin and into the river. My Stanford fraternity brother Ray Collis and I were donkey packing over Black Rock Pass in the late fall of 1957 and got caught in an early winter snow storm spending the night with our donkeys hunkered down behind rocks in the snow and rain in a full out winter storm.

I had a memorable experience in the upper Kern Canyon that I often look back upon. We had camped on the west bank of the river near Big Kern Lake and I was sitting out on a rock in the early morning savoring a hot cup of coffee. By about 10:30 a.m. the sun had summitted the eastern ridges of the Sierras and was penetrating down into the bottom of the Kern Canyon and as the bright summer sun made its way down the canyon walls it suddenly lit up the brilliant new green leaves of the aspen, cottonwood and willow trees on the river banks in an electrifying burst of color, stunning to behold in its beauty. I remained on the rock savoring the beauty of the moment.

In 1959 I hooked up with my friend John Rachford, a Stanford classmate who had been a summer packer for several seasons at the Mineral King Pack Station. Since this was John's last year and he was going to attend graduate school he was allowed to take two horses and a mule for a week long pack trip into the high Sierras. John invited me to join him and I readily agreed. John was an excellent horseman and packer and on the week-long trip I learned how to expertly tie a diamond hitch on the back of a pack mule. We packed out of Mineral King over Franklin Pass down Rattlesnake Canyon and leisurely explored the river camping in places off trail that John was aware of through his packing experiences. We took turns preparing meals on open firers over a grill, caught some good fish and saw a good deal of fantastic country. We took a tent but the weather was mild and we slept on our pads without a tent. It was a wonderful trip that I look back on fondly. It was a real cowboy experience.

From the Johnsondale Bridge I have hiked and fished the banks of the river down to Kernville. In the lower Kern Canyon I have fished much of it from Lake Isabella westward through Hobo Hot Springs, Delonga Hot Springs, Democrat Hot Springs and many points west along the river accessible by way of State Highway 178, the Kern Canyon Highway.

As a teenager one of my favorite fishing holes was the outlet at Cottonwood Creek into the river near Rancheria Bridge east of Bakersfield. This was a fishing opportunity that I partook in on many afternoons after school and on weekends with my high school fishing buddies Rusty Loman, Fred Perry and Bobby Carberry catching many fine trout at this hole where the Cottonwood Creek empties into the river. On one afternoon fishing expedition I ran into and had a face-off with a mountain lion who lived in the creek canyon.

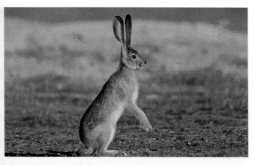
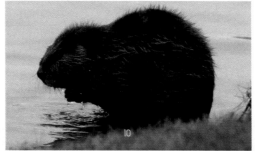
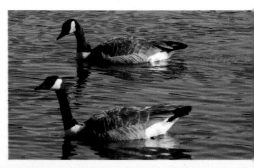

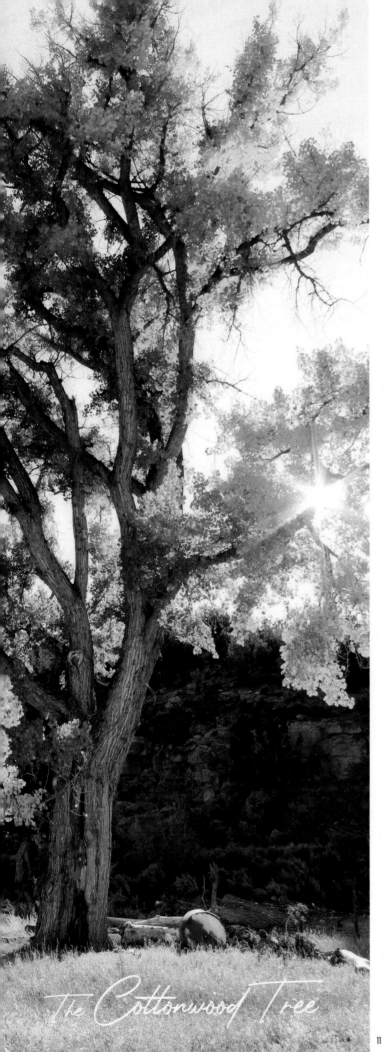

The Cottonwood Tree

As a teenager my gang and I frequently took raft trips on army surplus rafts from the mouth of the canyon on the river to Hart Park - a very dangerous but exhilarating white water rafting experience. I kayak the river frequently from Rancheria Bridge to Gordon's Ferry. I think I can say without exaggeration that I know as much about the Kern River, at least its geographics, as anyone.

Living on the river as I do now inevitably causes one to focus their attention on the cycles, the ebbs and flows and the currents of the river. From the beginning of the river at Lake South America at over 11,000 feet the river drops over 5,000 feet in the 180 miles to the San Joaquin Valley down to my house at 600 feet, one of the most precipitous drops of any river in the country. The Kern's river flows are exquisitely beautiful in its eddies swirls and upwellings.

In the twenty plus years I have lived on the banks of the river I daily monitor the flow of the river, particularly the CFS or the cubic feet per second of the river flow. CFS is an accepted measuring device to measure the flow of water. CFS is the amount of cubic feet of water that passes a measuring point in one second. A cubic foot of water is equivalent to 7.4 gallons of water. So if the CFS by my house is 1,000 CFS then this means there is approximately 7,400 gallons of water passing my house in one second. At 5,000 CFS a heavy flow in the spring with snow melt and runoff from the Sierras there would be 37,000 gallons of water passing the house each second. With a drop of 5,000 feet from its beginnings at Lake South America and 37,000 gallons per second coming out of the mouth of the river at the Kern Canyon as it empties into the San Joaquin Valley it is not difficult to understand why the river is so dangerous and the current so swift for an inexperienced swimmer or wader.

By watching the weather reports of accumulated snowfall in the Sierra Nevadas during the winter and spring one can get a good idea of what type of flow is going to be coming down the river in the spring and summer. From Mt. Whitney south the runoff in the Sierra Nevadas from the rain and snow melt into the Kern River Basin is both from the north fork and the south fork of the Kern River. The two forks - north and south - join up near the village of Onyx where both flow into Lake Isabella which has a capacity of 568,000 acre feet of water. Some of the runoff from the central Sierra does drains into the Kaweah River and Kings River Basins. From Thousand Island Lakes north of Mammoth the snow melt drains into the San Joaquin River Basin which exits the Sierras and is captured initially at Lake Millerton. The San Joaquin River exits Millerton Lake and eventually flows north through Fresno, Stockton into the Delta merging with the Sacramento River and into the San Francisco Bay

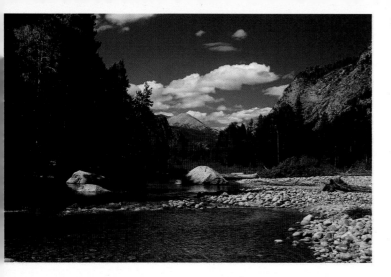

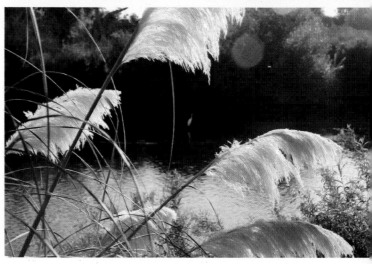

and eventually out under the Golden Gate to the Pacific Ocean. The Kern River, once it exits the Kern Canyon, flows into the San Joaquin Valley. From its exit from the mountains into the valley it enters a largely dry arid valley with a dessert climate. The southern San Joaquin Valley is largely a fertile farm area because of the water flows into the valley from the Kern, Kaweah, Kings and San Joaquin Rivers. The Kern Friant canal and the California Aqueduct also contribute water to the southern San Joaquin Valley agriculture bringing water from the Yuba River in northern California.

From its exit at the Kern Canyon into the valley and for 20 miles into Bakersfield the river is a life-sustaining corridor for the fauna and flora that live along its banks. Normally there is flowing water even in dry years from the mouth of the canyon down the riverbed for approximately 20 miles to where the river is divided into the Beardsley Canal and the Carrier Canal and diverted north and south in other canals for agricultural purposes. The river only flows through the city of Bakersfield in exceptionally wet years particularly when there is an above average snow fall in the Sierra Nevadas. People driving on Highway 99 cross the Kern River at Bakersfield, but in a dry year see only a dry riverbed. Little do they know that just 10 miles to the east is a substantial flow of water in the riverbed which is then diverted into canals for agricultural purposes and does not run through the city.

At my house the river never runs dry and we have water year round.

The historic end of the Kern River was at Buena Vista Lake near Taft where I used to duck hunt as a youth, but since the construction of the California Aqueduct the river now drains into the aqueduct intertie. The Aqueduct now transports the Kern River water to Southern California. Before the construction of the intertie in wet years the river could historically flow north through the central valley slough into the Tulare Lake basin and eventually into the San Joaquin River and then into San Francisco Bay. In abnormally wet years people from Bakersfield have made the trip by boat from Bakersfield to the end of the river then north on the Central Valley slough into Tulare Lake basin and into the San Joaquin River and eventually into San Francisco Bay. In my stories I describe kayaking from Bakersfield to the end of the river at the intertie.

I frequently kayak the river from the Kern River Golf Course to just above the Gordon Ferry Bridge on China Grade Loop Road, a distance of approximately 10 miles. The river through this stretch is excellent for kayaking particularly in the spring with good depths, swift current, minor rapids and beautiful riparian forest on both the north and south banks alive with a variety of bird life.

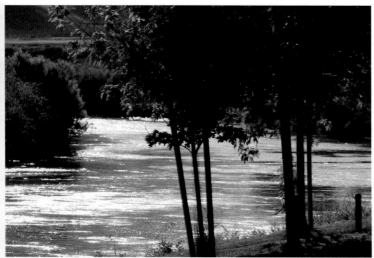

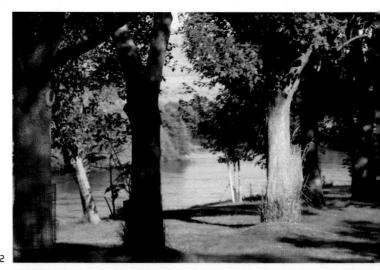

Sitting low in a kayak one cannot see anything other than the lush riparian forest along the banks and can concentrate on the varied bird life along the river. It is difficult to comprehend that just a few miles from a major city but so immersed in beautiful river life.

The critters that visit my property on the river are bears, mountain lions, coyotes, bobcats, raccoons, squirrels, skunks, possums, rabbits, deer, snakes - primarily king and rattle snakes - and an immense variety of insects and birds, ducks and geese and turtles and industrial sized bull frogs.

The bird life is extensive, and I help propagate it by providing nesting boxes for wood ducks and bird feeders for a variety of birds.

Regular bird visitors on my property are the giant blue herons, giant and lesser egrets, cormorants, eagles, peregine falcons, buzzards, hawks, kestrals and a great variety of ducks. The ducks are primarily seasonal although the mallards and the wood ducks will remain most of the year. Seasonal ducks are the buffleheads, Mergansers, Teal and occasional other visitors including a variety of diving ducks. The Canadian honkers are frequent fall and winter visitors to the property. They like to dive down in the water and gather the moss that grows on the bottom of the river when the water is shallow enough. They usually come back yearly for this treat. Other than the ducks there is a diverse bird life including finches of all varieties particularly the American canary, a finch that turns yellow during the mating season of January, February and March. Spring brings an invasion of blue jays, juncos, woodpeckers, flickers, black birds, blue birds, robins, king fishers and a variety of doves that remain throughout the year.

The hot dry San Joaquin Valley with its extensive agricultural production and abundant water supply is an ideal habitat for doves. The morning dove is the most common of the species, but the Eurasian collared dove is also very prevalent. There are also many bandtail pigeons which are often mistaken for doves. The relationship habits of the doves are fascinating. They engage in bowing and cooing as both a mating ritual and interrelationship ritual. The cooing of the doves in the late afternoon is a pleasing sound.

At my house on the river we have a healthy population of doves because of the ideal habitat: water, feed and abundant locations for nesting in the trees along the river. From my deck on the edge of the river I have a collection of binoculars where I can observe the comings and goings of many of the these feathered creatures.

One of my favorite birds on the river is the wood duck that in my opinion is one of the most beautiful of all nature's birds. I write about my association with this beautiful creature in one of the chapters of this book. Both the wood duck drake and hen are permanent visitors to my property during the mating season because I do provide nesting boxes for the hens and usually see anywhere from thirty to forty new wood ducklings hatching each year.

I also have a colony of beavers that live just across the river deck where I can closely observe their comings and goings. They were originally a nuisance when I first moved in as they were chewing down my hedges and trees. I have since learned to put rabbit wire around all of my trees near the water's edge as well as my hedges to protect them from being taken down by the beavers. The beavers and I have managed to coexist with one another for some time. One old patriarch beaver who lives in the den across the river is so large that I liken him to a small bear. He can certainly startle you with a flap of his tail on the water before he submerges.

I also like to watch the comings and goings of the giant egrets and blue herons who usually feed on the banks in the shallow water when the flow is down. There is a small clam that lives in the river and both the herons and egrets like to clam in the sandy banks at low river. In addition to the clams the herons and egrets are good fishermen and harvest small fish from the river's edges.

The fish in the river are trout, bass, bluegill, whitefish and catfish. The whitefish grow to a substantial size as well as the catfish. My nephew Gino Valpredo and his son Nicco who live up the river from me frequently fish the river with their fishing tubes casting out for fish.

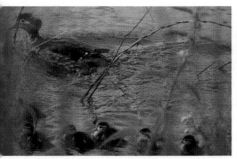
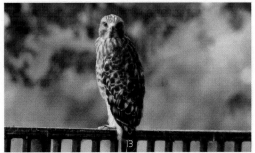
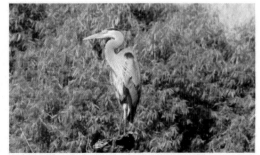

A daily visitor to my property is the racoons. The river-banks are full of insects, lizards, birds, duck eggs and other goodies that the raccoons love to feast on. The banks along both sides of the river I call the raccoon turnpike as they are always on the move east and west along the riverbanks. Some are quite large.

Coyotes are frequent visitors. There is a pack of coyotes on the south bank and a distinct pack of coyotes on the north bank. Sometimes in the early evenings the two packs will howl and bark back and forth at one another across the river. The river prevents them from crossing, but they carry on a lively exchange of barking and howling which my wife and I refer to as the coyote symphony. The coyotes' howling excites my cocker spaniels who join in with their own howling. Our dogs are protected from coyotes by a wrought iron fence.

My wife recounts one evening where she was working at her desk by the window when a mountain lion sauntered down the walkway from the entrance to the house, glanced at my wife and casually kept moving down the walkway to the driveway. Deer will occasionally pass by munching on the fresh green grass in the spring and sometimes eating ripe apples off the trees.

I have a flock of green parrots who visit my orchard like clockwork in the late spring to eat all of my newly ripened cherries. They seem to have an inner sense of time as to just when the cherries are at the peak of their sweetness.

We had a den of bobcats living along the river for a number of years. They are beautiful creatures who do well with the abundance of squirrels and rabbits in the area.

The flora along the river which also depends on the water for its existence is immense and varied. Over the generations the nature of the flora along the riparian edges of the stream has evolved. The mainstays are the giant California sycamores and cottonwoods and willows that can grow to immense sizes in the rich riverbed soil. A protected species of plant that flourishes along the river is the elderberry, a bush-like tree that produces a beautiful white flowers and purple elderberries in the fall that the birds crave.

One of the most beautiful benefits to living on the Kern River is to be able to monitor its constantly changing moods and manifestations throughout the year. In the spring the river can be a rushing torrent channeling a swirling current of snow melt rain and runoff from hundreds of miles of the high Sierras. This high water level often reaching 5,000 CFS can alter the flora along the banks of the river by taking out dead wood, weak trees, older bushes and changing the channel of the river. The cat tails that flourish during the summer months are often ripped out changing the habitat of bird life and fish. In the summer the long days and evenings can bring a series of dramatic sunsets. As the sun disappears behind the coastal range the river surface can turn to silver, merge into pink and gold depending upon the alpenglow glow in the west and then gradually disappear into darkness as the light from the western sky disappears. Every sunset is different and unique. In the winter autumn trees along the banks take on their fall colors which adds another dramatic aspect to the river channel. In the winter when the high water recedes and the river becomes more peaceful and slow moving and restful the ducks can swim easily up current. Being on the water can evoke a sense of awe and magic - a feeling of calm. I often remark to visitors that when I travel out Round Mountain Road toward my home passing the last curve where I descend down into the river basin my blood pressure recedes and a feeling of calmness and peace pervades.

In the front yard of my river house there is an ancient cottonwood tree of enormous size. An arborist who examined the tree estimates its age as probably 150 years old. Under the shaded branches of this tree would have been an ideal place to camp-shady, flat ground with good grass, and good water just a few feet away. I realize that where I live has been an attractive place to "camp" for many years, probably eons. In 1776 Father Francisco Garces, a Franciscan missionary, named the river Rio de San Felipe. Father Garces according to his accounts crossed the river in 1776 about 10 miles east of my house. The name of the river was changed in August 1806 by Padre Zavida, a Spanish explorer, who renamed the river La Porciuncula for the day of the Porciuncula indulgence. The local Indians called the river the Po-Sun-Co-La, a derivation of Porciuncula. In 1845 John Fremont named the river for Edward M. Kern, his topographer, on his third expedition through the American west. Kern narrowly escaped drowning while attempting to cross the river.

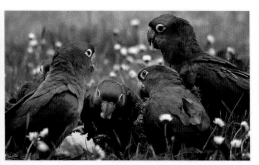
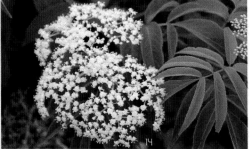
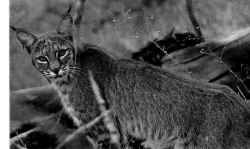

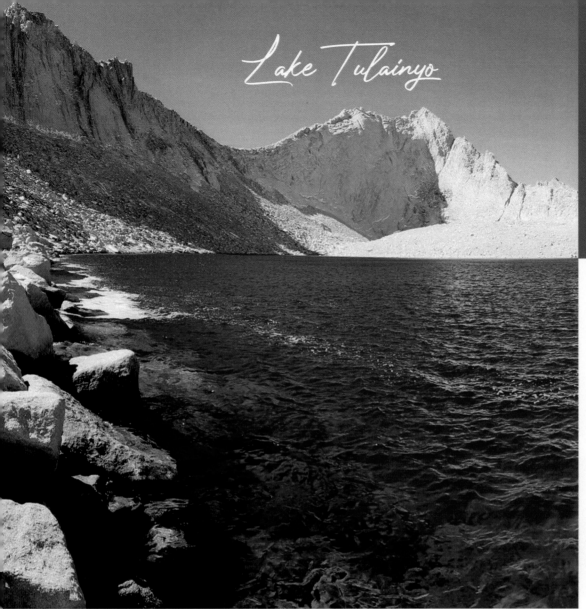

Lake Tulainyo

Native people have been known to live along the Po-Sun-Co-La as early as 100 A.D. and may have lived here even earlier. The river has been a vital lifeline for humans and animals for thousands of years. John Muir wrote in his book The Yosemite that "...everybody needs beauty as well as bread, places to play in and pray in, where nature may heal and give strength to the body and soul alike." The Kern is such a place.

THE PO-SUN-CO-LA
... has given me the opportunity to live a life in beauty ...

I have always been fascinated by The Navajos and the Anasazi concept of living one's life in beauty. These indigenous people have lived on this earth for centuries and have developed a concept of life which is embodied in the Navajo phrase "Walking in Beauty". To walk in beauty is to live one's life absorbed in the beauty of life, the beauty of life above in the sky, the clouds, the wind, the moon, sun, stars, rain, snow, storms; the beauty of the forest, trees, and the intricate beauty of flowers; the beauty of the creatures of the earth who share this small planet with us.

The sense of living life in beauty is expressed in excerpts from the Navajo Blessing Way Prayer

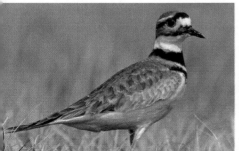
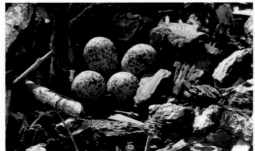
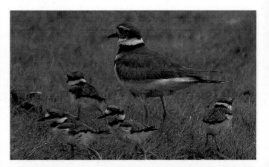

15

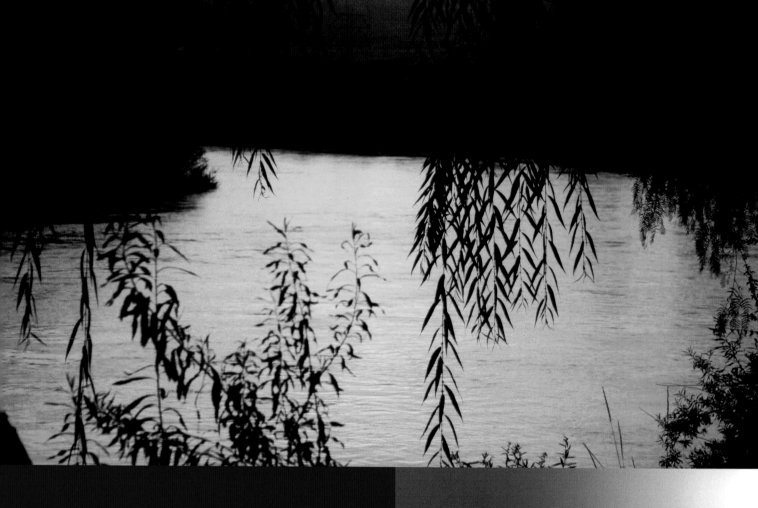

Navajo Way Blessing

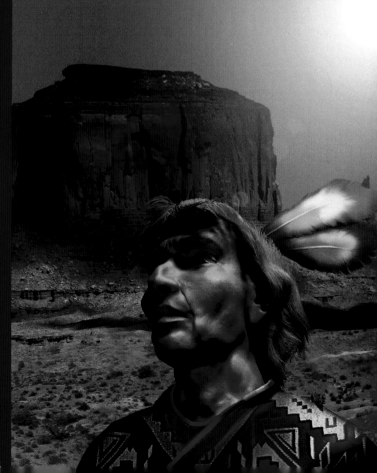

With beauty before me, I walk.
With beauty behind me, I walk.
With beauty below me, I walk.
With beauty above me, I walk.
With beauty all around me, I walk.

In old age wandering on a trail of beauty,
lively, may I walk.

In old age wandering on a trail of beauty,
living again, may I walk.

It is finished in beauty.
It is finished in beauty.
It is finished in beauty.

Excerpts from the closing prayer of the
Navajo Way Blessing Ceremony.

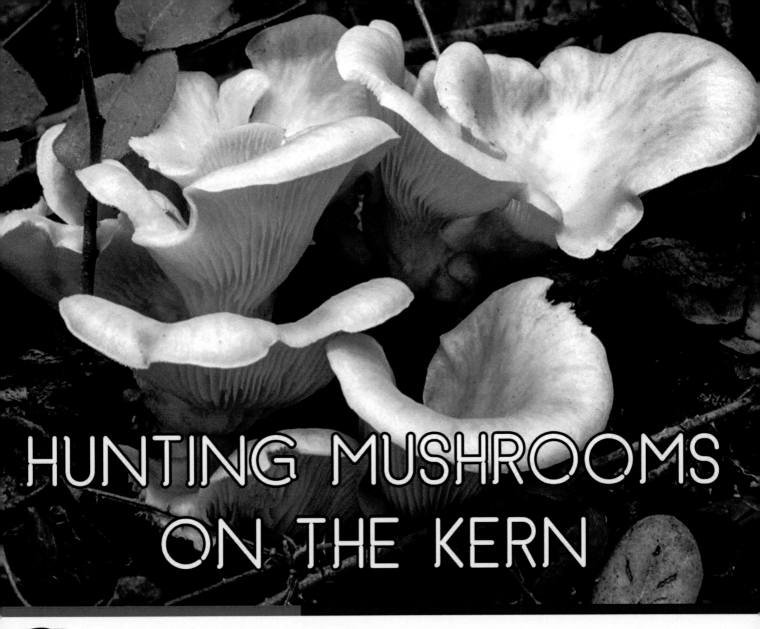

HUNTING MUSHROOMS ON THE KERN

One of the reasons I fell in love with the Kern River at an early age was my childhood trips to the river bottom to search for tree mushrooms. I must have been five or six years old when I began accompanying my father, a mushroom connoisseur, on his river bottom forages for tree mushrooms. The Kern River bottom lands, especially east of the Beardsley Weirs below the bluffs, were a paradise for tree mushroom lovers. The best season was usually late winter/early spring, particularly after a wet winter season. Also the heavy fogs that we used to have in the San Joaquin Valley were ideal growing-conditions for the tree mushrooms. Most of our mushroom hunting trips were conducted along the north and south banks of the Kern River at the bottom of China Grade. In those days usually the willow and cottonwood trees were the best hosts for the tree mushrooms. There were also giant syca-mores, a native California species, that could grow to a considerable height that hosted the tree mushrooms.

My father and my grandfather knew the mushrooms that we were looking for by sight. They did not need a book or photograph to identify the mushroom. The tree mushroom that we looked for and harvested was the Pleurotus Ostreatus, also referred to as oyster mushrooms. In California this tree mushroom can be found varying from white and relatively thin-fleshed on oak trees to thick-fleshed gray brown shelves on cottonwood and willow trees. We found them mostly on the cottonwood and willow trees, particularly in areas of the trees that had deteriorated and rotted.

My father usually supplied me with a bucket with my name on it. Later on I was given a sharp knife to carefully separate the tree mushroom fungus from the trees. The knife hung from a strap on the bucket. It was only after I learned to use the knife safely that I had my own.

The area below the bluffs was heavily forested in those days with the willows, cottonwoods and underlying brush. This area could usually only be penetrated by animals or hobos, but my father knew the routes that would lead us down to the river. These were usually hobo trails that led to their encampments. The hobos never bothered us, and we did not bother them.

Another of our familiar spots to hunt for mushrooms was along Poso Creek - about one mile east of the Granite / Glenville Road off Poso Creek Road.

My father had a knack which he carried for his life of just knowing when to search for the mushrooms. If it was too dry and not enough rain or moisture or fog had been in the weather pattern the mushrooms would not have sprouted out of their host trees. Pop knew just the best times to search for the mushrooms and most likely developed that characteristic from his father, Joe Lemucchi, who also hunted mushrooms along the river bottom from the early 1900's.

We would drive down China Grade Loop Road, exit onto a dirt road down into the area where the Gun Club was located or where the Shell refinery is now located and park and then take the hobo trails down along the river.

We would spend the morning combing through the river bottom looking for the fungus around the big cottonwood, willow and sycamore trees.

The tree mushrooms that we harvested had medium to large size caps and very short or none existent stems. The caps are broad and fan-like ranging in color from dark gray, pinkish and have curled edges. White gills extend from beneath the cap and the flesh is white, meaty and firm. The mushrooms have a slightly chewy texture. The mushrooms are found growing on decaying wood as indicated in the river bottom on sycamores, cottonwood and willows. These mushrooms are extremely popular and there are many knowledgeable mushroom hunters in Kern County which means that you have to get out and hunt for them when the conditions are right.

Tree mushrooms are native to North America and have been growing wild since ancient times.

After we picked buckets of tree mushrooms we would load them into the back of my dad's Jeep station wagon and deliver the mushrooms to the kitchen at Lemucchi's Grocery Store on East 19th Street for preparation. My father filled the wash tubs with water, poured in the freshly picked mushrooms and gave them a good bath. He would then put them in colanders to drain.

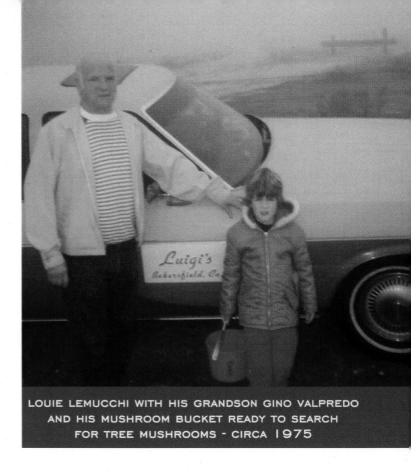

LOUIE LEMUCCHI WITH HIS GRANDSON GINO VALPREDO AND HIS MUSHROOM BUCKET READY TO SEARCH FOR TREE MUSHROOMS - CIRCA 1975

My father continued our family tradition of searching for tree mushrooms when he continued to take the next generation of the family, his grandchildren: Lisa, Monica, Lanette and Gino on hunts with him. Each grandchild had their own painted bucket with their name on the side. The grand kids, now grown adults in their 50s, fondly recall the river mushroom excursions and still relish eating Emelia's prepared tree mushrooms.

After the mushrooms had dried off my dad and grandmother would cut them into thin strips, one-half inch wide and two to three inches long.

The fungi then would be placed in large jars filled with my grandfather's special brine. The mushrooms would soak in the brine until such time as they were ready to be consumed. Garlic cloves and oregano "cured" in the brine, and after a couple of weeks the mushrooms would be ready for consumption.

They could be eaten raw about thirty days after they were "cured" in the raw.

Tree mushrooms are the best and are excellent in stir-fries, pasta, lasagna and pizza. Tree mushrooms cook relatively quickly and are typically added at the end of the cooking process. They are popularly used in many Asian dishes - in Japanese, Korean and Chinese cuisine. They can also be dried for extended use and do not have to be re-hydrated before using.

They pair well with onions, shallots, green onions, garlic, ginger, potatoes, thyme, parsley, peas, green beans, eggplant, poultry, lemon and spaghetti.

My favorite recipe, however, was when my grandmother, Emelia Lemucchi, prepared fried mushroom strips. Emelia's recipe was to remove the fungi from the brine and let them dry on paper towels. She would then dip them in egg batter and roll them in flour. She would then lightly fry them in olive oil and garlic until slightly crisp on the outside but spongy and hot in the center. She would place them on towels on a platter to drain, lightly sprinkle with lemon juice and serve them hot or warm. Talk about delicious! This was the best reward for the mushroom hunt. Fried mushrooms were a delicacy we could count on for Christmas, Thanksgiving and other holidays.

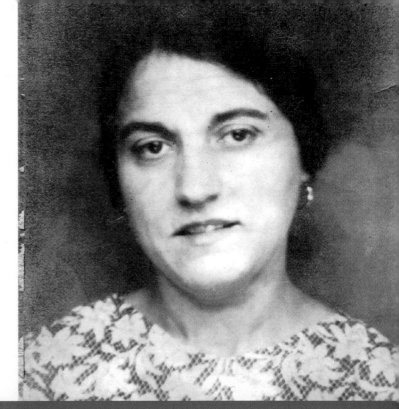

MY GRANDMOTHER, EMELIA LEMUCCHI

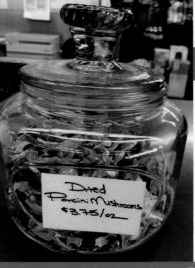

Dried Porcini Mushrooms $3.75/oz

Luigi's
BAKERSFIELD, CA.
SERVING FAMILY AND FRIENDS SINCE 1910
LEMUCCHI-VALPREDO

"MY FAVORITE RECIPE, WAS WHEN MY GRANDMOTHER, EMELIA LEMUCCHI, PREPARED FRIED MUSHROOM STRIPS"

TO THIS DAY LUIGI'S OLD WORLD DELICATESSEN IN BAKERSFIELD, CALIFORNIA CONTINUES THE TRADITION

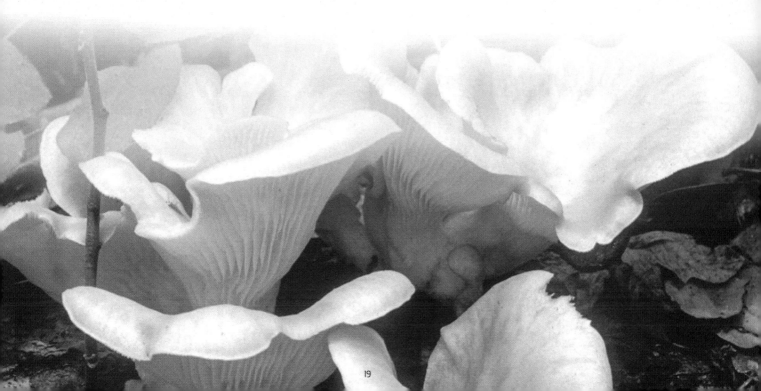

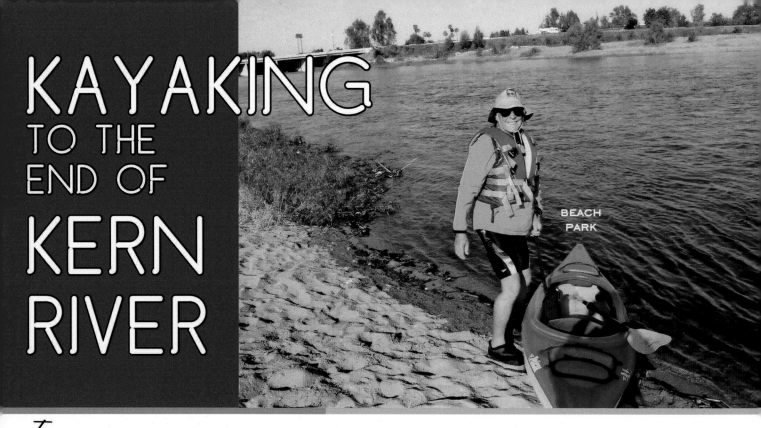

BEACH
PARK

KAYAKING
TO THE
END OF
KERN
RIVER

It requires an unusually wet winter or a decision by the U.S. Corps of Army dam engineers to release surplus water from Lake Isabella for water to flow the length of the Kern River. The winter and spring of the year 2011 was a convergence of both conditions, resulting in one of the greatest recreational adventure opportunities in the arid southern San Joaquin Valley.

With the Sierrra Nevada winter snow pack 190 % of its normal and water engineers forced to keep Lake Isabella at 60 % of its capacity for structural safety reasons an unusual amount of water was cascading down the Kern Canyon to Bakersfield and the San Joaquin Valley. It was an adventure that could not be missed.

Before Bakersfield became a major city, the river flowed through swampland. Elisha Stephens, an early Kern County pioneer came through the area in 1844 on his way to San Diego. He described the swampland, which is now Bakersifeld's core, as a forest of cotton-wood, willows, elder and sycamore trees. The Kern River was named for Edward Meyer Kern (1823-1863), a draftsman topographer with John C. Freemont's expedition to the west. Freemont noted in his journals that the river was known to native Califor-nians as the Po-Sun-Co-La. But nearly a century later, when Father Francisco Garces traveled through the area, he called it the Rio San Felipe and described it as having "waters crystalline, bountiful and palatable ."

Before the Lake Isabella Dam was built in the 1960s heavy spring runoffs from snow melt poured water down

the Kern River into the valley flooding Bakersfield, Buena Vista Lake and much of the southwest valley floor quite frequently. The river flowed southward into Buena Vista Lake which covered thousands of acres, and in very wet years would backup if more, and overflow into a series of sloughs that would drain into the Tulare Lake and then into the San Joaquin River where it would travel to the San Francisco Bay and the Pacific Ocean. The 353 mile route from its origins high in the eastern Sierra made it one of the longer river systems in California. In the past Kern County residents have taken boats from Bakersfield to the end of the river and through the slough channels into the San Joaquin drainage and out to San Francisco Bay.

The dam was built in 1966 to control the rivers's flow and store water for regulated delivery to farmers. A decade later the California Aqueduct was built. The old river bed at its end was channeled into an intertie which empties into the California Aqueduct sending Kern River waters southward to the Edmonston Pumping Plant and over the Tehachapi Mountains into southern California and eventually into the ocean. With the dam's construction also came a myriad of weirs and canals, diverting the water for irrigation of farmland. This diversion caused the stream bed below its diversion into weirs and canals to become dry and sandy except in unusually wet years.

In the year 2006, also an unusually wet year, Bakers-field contractor Steve Prasser, civil engineer Terry Shroepfer and I kayaked to the river's end. To cele-brate the Kern River's spectacular rebirth in the year 2011 we recreated our earlier trip.

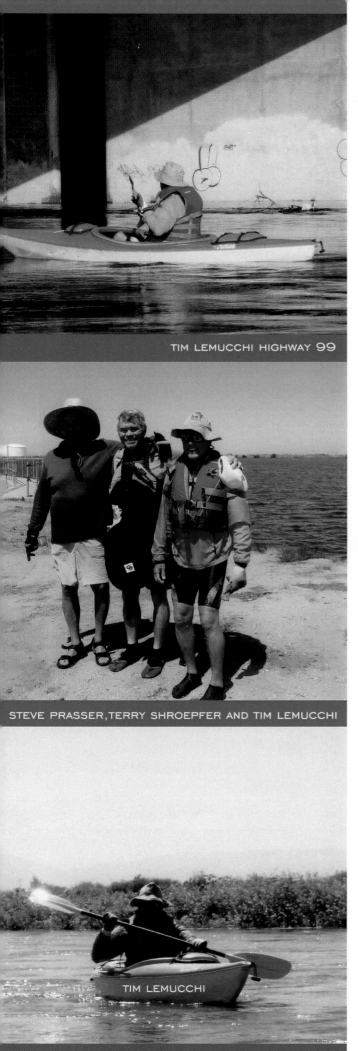

TIM LEMUCCHI HIGHWAY 99

STEVE PRASSER, TERRY SHROEPFER AND TIM LEMUCCHI

TIM LEMUCCHI

We launched our kayaks at 8:00 a.m. from Beach Park on April 30, 2011 and arrived at the river's end six and a half hours later. The water level and current flow to the river's end were excellent. We never scraped the kayaks' bottoms on rocks and never hung up on sand bars.

Evidence of dry years between 2006 and 2011 could be seen on the riverbanks from Beach Park to Allen Road. Many of the established aquatic plants, the old cottonwoods and willows had died. Their leafless skeletal remains dotted the bank. The vegetation on the riverbanks that had survived the drought provided habitat for abundant bird and animal life.

We saw fewer birds in 2011 than in 2006. In 2006 there was an abundance of grebs, white pelicans, cormorants, bitterns, great blue herons, great egrets, snowy egrets, green herons, white-faced ibis, mergansers, stilts, avocets and a large population of ducks, mostly mallards.

One of the most interesting parts of the river was found west of Allen Road where you can easily imagine that you have returned to what the river looked like 200 years ago. Instead of the hundreds of birds we encountered in 2011, two hundred years ago there were hundreds of thousands of birds as well as wildlife that included mountain lions, ringtail cats, coyotes, bobcats, badgers, foxes, bears, antelope, deer and elk. The area is now populated with rabbits, quail, roadrunners, snakes, squirrels, raccoons, skunks and other species that depend upon the river for water.

Kayaking under Enos Lane beyond the bridge we entered a fascinating swampland. The high flow of the river had only recently come through this area and the new river channel was not yet well established. There were many plants and bushes protruding up through the water giving the appearance of an everglades-type swampland. The channel was not always clear, but if one followed the main current and paddled around the protruding vegetation it could be navigated.

The area below Interstate 5 was completely isolated and removed from any signs of civilization. It appeared so remote but was only a few miles west of Bakersfield.

In 1987 the Kern River was added by Congress to the National Wild and Scenic River System.

From its beginnings at Lake South America at over 11,400 feet in the eastern Sierras near Mt. Whitney, the Kern River plunges thousands of feet into the Kern Canyon carving its way through solid rock and dividing its flow around huge boulders before emptying out into the verdant San Joaquin Valley. The Kern River is truly one of California's most beautiful and impressive river systems. My friends and I had the privilege of experiencing this unique water system.

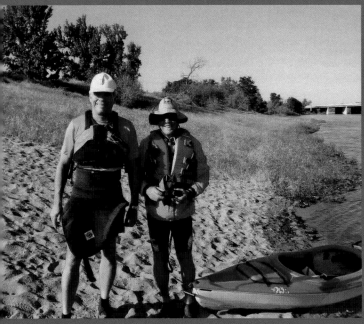

TERRY SHROEPFER & TIM LEMUCCHI

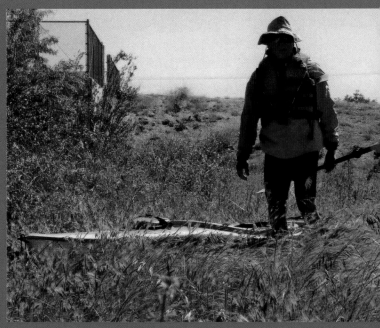

READY TO EXPERIENCE THIS UNIQUE WATER SYSTEM

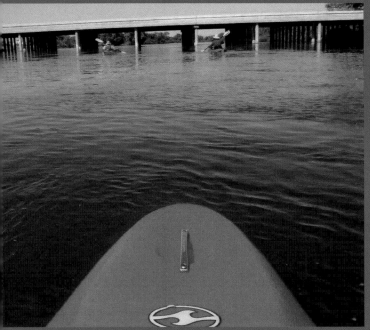

APPROACHING CALLOWAY BRIDGE

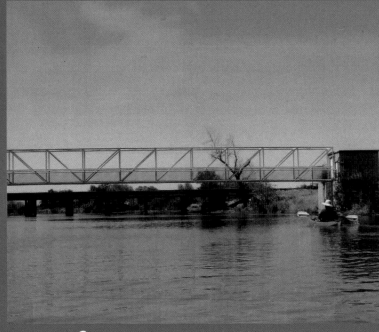

2ND POINT - WEST OF ENOS LANE

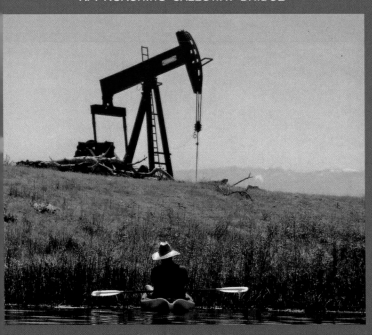

STEVE PRASSER

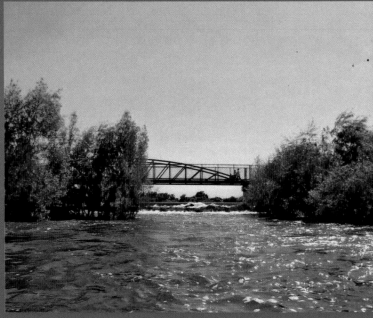

2ND PORTAGE - BIKE BRIDGE AT RIVER PARK

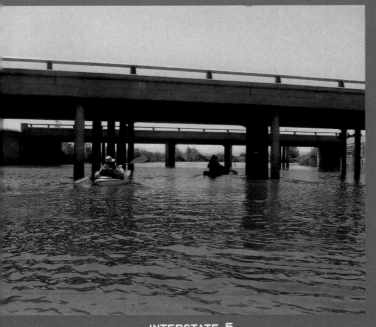

INTERSTATE 5
NORMALLY DRY AND SAND UNDERNEATH

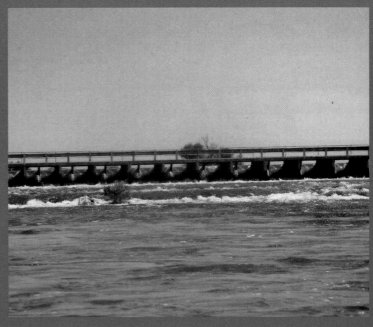

MCCLUNG WEIR DOWNSTREAM AFTER PORTAGE

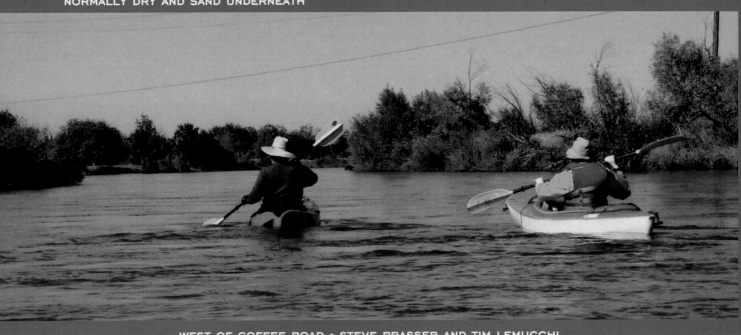

WEST OF COFFEE ROAD - STEVE PRASSER AND TIM LEMUCCHI

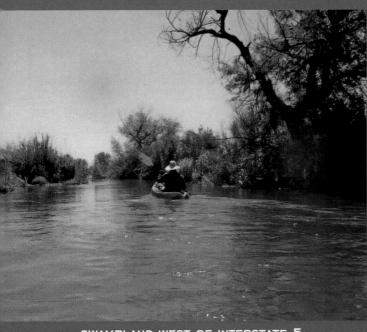

SWAMPLAND WEST OF INTERSTATE 5

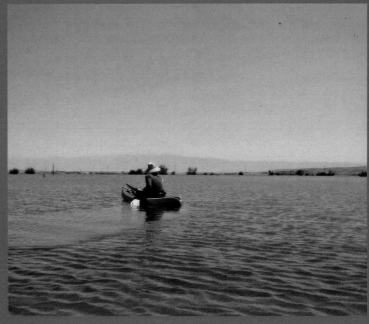

LARGE LAKE - END OF RIVER AT AQUEDUCT INTER-TIE

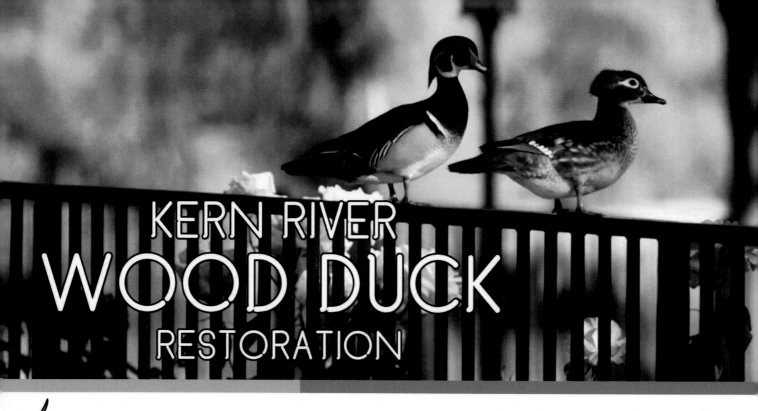

KERN RIVER WOOD DUCK RESTORATION

Living on the Kern River as I have now for many years I have become fascinated with the duck life at my doorstep. My river patio sits a few feet above the water's edge, and I have spent many hours with a hot cup of coffee in the morning or a glass of Pinot Noir in the late afternoon watching the comings and goings of my feathered friends: the mallard, the wood duck, the bobble head, the teal, the mergansers and also the herons, giant egrets and the myraid of other birds that frequent the riparian forest of the river. I have become particularly fascinated by the wood duck.

Once threatened with near extinction one of California's most beautiful waterfowl is making a comeback in the San Joaquin Valley. In the late 1800s and early 1900s extinction of the wood duck was described as imminent. Destruction of bottom land forest, draining of swamps, ponds and lakes and market hunting were major causes of the birds' decline. Thanks to some farsighted environmental management, hunting regulations and citizen volunteers the wood duck is making a welcome comeback.

Many people feel that the male wood duck is one of the most beautiful of all of nature's birds. The markings of a male drake wood duck include red eyes and a red bill with a yellow patch at the base. The top of the bird's head and crest is a metallic purplish green. On the side of the face is a black and white stripe that runs around the neck. A small white stripe also extends up each cheek. The chest and the rear are dark red. The sides are a drab yellow with black and white stripes at the edges. The drake's belly is white, its tail and back are black and its

wings are black and blue. If you have ever had the opportunity to view a drake wood duck up close or through binoculars, particularly on a bright sunny day, its image is striking.

The drake's colorful markings are especially brilliant during the breeding season which runs from autumn until early summer. They use their colorful markings to attract females.

The female wood duck is also quite distinctive. They have grayish brown bodies with their sides being a lighter shade. The most noticeable feature of the hen or female is the head which is gray with a white ring around each eye that gives the female a rather exotic look.

Approximately 75% of the wood ducks found in California in the Pacific flyway are non-migratory.

The southern San Joaquin Valley was historically an ideal habitat for the wood duck, and populations were substantial.

The wood ducks' ideal habitat is wooded swamps, shallow lakes, marshes or ponds, creeks and rivers. They would usually nest in tree cavities close to the water. The lower San Joaquin Valley which - historically was largely flooded wetlands - was an ideal habitat.

The population of the wood duck as indicated was in serious decline in the late nineteenth century as a result of severe habitat loss and market hunting both for meat and plumage for ladies' hats marketed in Europe.

In response to the Migratory Bird Treaty established in 1916 and the enactment of the U.S. Migratory Bird Treaty Act of 1918 wood duck populations began to recover slowly. Also during this time the southern end of the San Joaquin Valley was being vigorously drained of its ponds, swamps and lakes and trees removed to make way for farming.

The southern end of the San Joaquin Valley, due to its wet marshlands, was also ideal habitat for large cotton-wood trees, willows and sycamores all of which provided woody cavities in which the ducks could nest and lay their eggs. In fact the wood duck was known as a cavity duck because it made its nest in cavities in trees close to water.

In addition to the Migratory Bird Treaties of 1916 and 1918, land owners as well as refuge managers and farmers, primarily beginning in the 1930s based on innovated practices from the eastern United States, did help restore wood duck populations by adding man-made nesting boxes to the banks of rivers, lakes and streams. The Kern River in particular has always been an optimal habitat for wood ducks.

In spite of the land clearing and swamp draining that went on in the lower valley, the streams that ran into the valley from the Sierras - the San Joaquin River, the Kern, the Tulare, the Kaweah, the Kings - usually had enough spring and summer snow melt runoff to help keep the riparian foliage growing. These streams did retain much of their natural bank foliage at least on the western slopes of the Sierras to include the important cavity-producing trees such as cottonwoods, willows and sycamores. Woodies usually prefer trees close to water. The females will line their nest with feathers and other soft materials. A higher elevation in the tree provides some protection from predators. The man-made boxes are usually filled with wood chips and/or moss to expedite cleaning.

Unlike most other ducks the wood duck has sharp claws on its feet for perching in trees. And the wood duck is one of the only ducks that can produce two broods in a single season.

Females typically lay between 7 to 15 white/tan eggs that incubate for about thirty days. After hatching the ducklings climb to the opening of the nest cavity and jump down from the tree nest to make their way to water. The mother will call them to her but does not help them in any way. Oftentimes it is quite a jump from the nest to the ground and then more distance to the shore and then water. The ducklings can swim immediately and find their own food by this time. They mainly eat berries, seeds, insects, tiny fish, crustaceans and other invertebrates. With the use of the man-made nesting box the little ducklings use their claws to climb up the inside of the nesting box and jump out the hole entrance sometimes 7 to 10 feet to the ground.

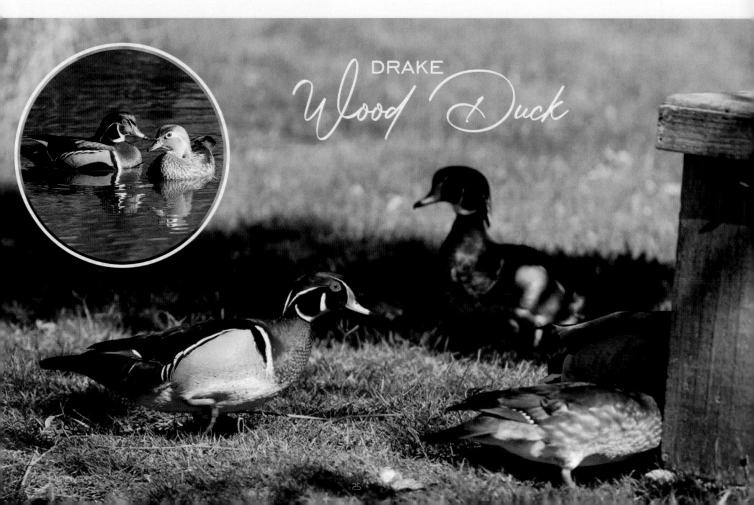

DRAKE
Wood Duck

There are many videos available on YouTube that show the ducklings' "jump day." These videos are a delight to watch, especially for young children. Even though the mothers do not help the ducklings they do fall in line behind her and it is an amazing and unforgettable sight to see 7 to 10 little ducklings swimming in line behind their mother in the river.

The Kern River as a wood duck hatchery has been supported by a number of volunteers who live in the valley and some who live on the river that provide nesting boxes on their property and take the responsibility for their maintenance and keeping them clean and out of the reach of predators.

Wood ducks have many predators: coyotes, snakes, skunks, racoons, foxes, hawks, bobcats and even large catfish and bass.

Much of the funding for the construction plans and placement of the artificial nesting boxes along the Kern River has been provided by the Tulare Lakes Basin Water Association (TBWA). Presently on the Kern River from the Manor Street bridge to Hart Park there are some forty-five hand-built nesting boxes on the north and south banks of the river.

People affiliated with TBWA use a hovercraft, a boat with a large wind-driven propeller, to carry the boxes up the river and place them.

During the high water on the Kern River of 2017, where the water was moving at times up to 5,000 cubic feet a second, some twenty nesting boxes were lost. Those have been restored.

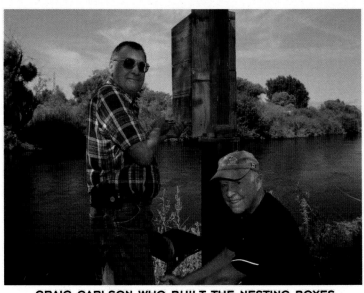

CRAIG CARLSON WHO BUILT THE NESTING BOXES
AND TIMOTHY LEMUCCHI

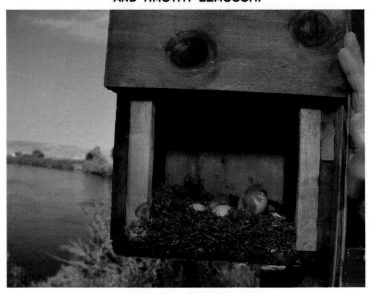

INTERIOR OF NESTING BOX
WITH DOOR OFF SHOWING WOOD DUCK EGGS

According to people who monitor the wood duck population the older and more mature birds will use the nest first, lay and hatch their eggs, and then the nests will be taken over by the younger birds. Although most of the birds in the San Joaquin Valley are non-migratory the birds do tend to move to Lake Isabella over the winter and return to the lower areas of the Kern beginning in March for the breeding season. The use of man-made nesting boxes along the Kern River has been in existence for approximately ten years.

They have proved their worth in substantially increasing the wood duck population in the Kern River drainage.

The use of man-made nesting boxes supports the position that farming, game management, and bird conservation can coexist, and the expanding wood duck population of this beautiful bird along the Kern River supports this coexistence.

TIMOTHY LEMUCCHI HAS LIVED ON THE NORTH BANK OF THE KERN RIVER FOR OVER FIFTEEN YEARS AND IN 2005 BEGAN INSTALLING FOUR NESTING BOXES ON HIS PROPERTY. TWO OF THE BOXES WERE WASHED OUT IN THE HIGH WATER OF 2017 WHERE WATER WAS RUNNING OVER 5,000 CFS. BUT SINCE 2005 LEMUCCHI USUALLY HAS WOOD DUCK HATCHES OF TWENTY-FIVE TO THIRTY-FIVE NEW DUCKLINGS A YEAR.

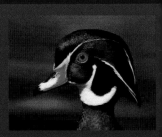

THE VERY SPECIAL HIGH SIERRA JEWEL
ROCK CREEK CABIN

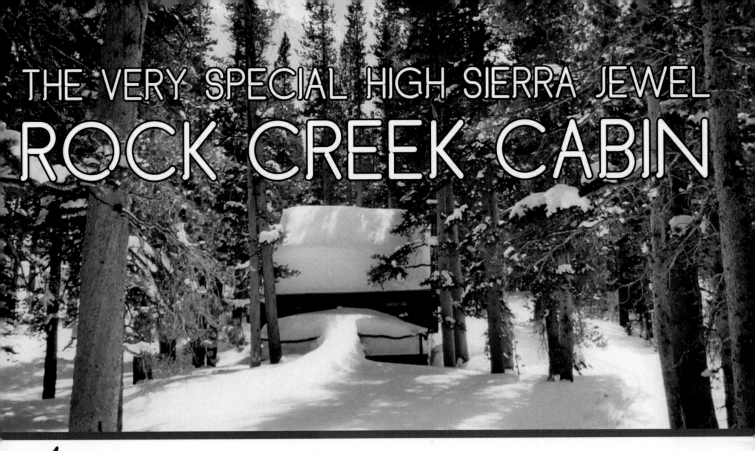

My ability to become very proficient at high sierra back country skiing and mountaineering is largely due to my involvement with a very special place in the high sierras - Rock Creek Cabin. Rock Creek Cabin sits on a forested bench at 10,000 feet in the eastern sierra.

The cabin at 10,000 feet, is 400 feet above Rock Creek Lake which is noted for its crystal blue waters. The area around the cabin is home to an abundant wildlife including black bears, mountains lions, mule deer, pine martin, pika and many species of birds. The lake and the streams in Rock Creek Canyon are full of rainbow trout.

The cabin is accessible in the summer by a rough road I call a goat trail that starts at a locked forest service gate at the Rock Creek campground and winds up over a rough, rocky, un-maintained road with an elevation gain of 600 feet to the cabin. In the winter the cabin is completely isolated, and the only access is by skis or snowshoes. Deep snow prevents one from walking to the cabin. In the winter access to the cabin is from the east fork campground on Rock Creek Road five miles from the cabin. The cabin is only about two miles from the John Muir wilderness and the Little Lakes basin, a string of high elevation lakes surrounded by 13,000 foot peaks including Bear Creek Spire at 13,100 feet. I became involved in the cabin in 1981 when I purchased an interest from Doug Robinson who had owned and rehabilitated the cabin.

The cabin was originally built in 1947 by Jack Kessler, a Hollywood cameraman, who built it himself on forest service lease land. Apparently he had a Dodge truck and hauled materials up the rocky road into the cabin in the summer. Kessler was known as a likeable, good-natured outdoors man. When he built the original cabin people told him that it would collapse in a heavy winter, which it did in the 1960s down to the loft floor.

Kessler's original cabin had four small rooms, two small bedrooms, one for a kitchen and one for a living area, with an upstairs loft for sleeping. Kessler rebuilt the cabin after snow weight collapsed it. In 1975 Doug Robinson purchased the cabin from Kessler and instead of re-doing the four rooms he opened up the interior to one larger downstairs room and put in a large beam to support the roof which was held up by two large tree poles. Robinson insulated the walls and the roof and substituted plate glass for seven enlarged window openings. He lined the interior with weathered barn boards and plastered the loft walls.

In 1981 Bob Tyson, AJ Marsden and I bought in as partners. Our original idea was to use the cabin as a base to explore the high elevation, Little Lakes Valley and ski the Bear Creek spire, the mountain that overlooks the giant cirque at the head of Rock Creek Canyon.

Norman Clyde, a famous sierra mountain man, called the Bear Creek Spire cirque the greatest skiing in the Sierras.

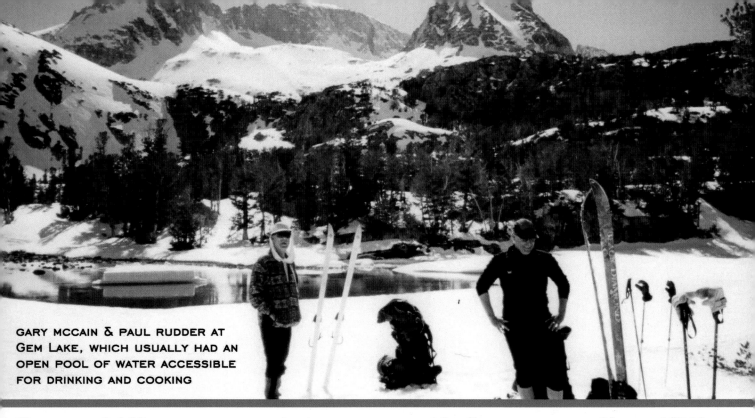

GARY MCCAIN & PAUL RUDDER AT
GEM LAKE, WHICH USUALLY HAD AN
OPEN POOL OF WATER ACCESSIBLE
FOR DRINKING AND COOKING

There are no chairlifts, rope tows on any other mechanical devices to get to the giant bowls of the Bear Creek Spire - the only way there in the winter is by human-powered skis.

The cabin in summer can be reached via Highway 395 at the turnoff to Tom's Place on the road to Mosquito Flats. From Tom's Place to Rock Creek Lake it is nine miles. From Tom's Place to Mosquito Flats, the highest road end in the eastern Sierra at 11,000 feet it is another three miles or a total of twelve, the last three miles on a narrow, bumpy, potholed filled road.

In the winter it was a nine mile ski from Tom's Place to Rock Creek Lake, then another mile to the cabin - a total of ten miles. That made for a long day with a heavy pack and a two thousand foot elevation gain.

Once the Forest Service started clearing snow from the Rock Creek road to the east Fork Campground in the early 1980s (about five miles) - the trip in the wintertime to the cabin became much easier. The elevation at the east fork of Rock Creek is about 8,000 feet so there was an additional 2,000 feet of climbing over five miles to reach the cabin. If you skied the road the elevation rise was gradual, but if you went up to Rock Creek trail there were some steep parts.

In 1981 after becoming involved in the cabin I took my daughter Lisa to the cabin in January. We parked the car at the east fork and took a snow mobile furnished by Rock Creek Winter Lodge from there into Rock Creek Winter Lodge. Rock Creek Winter Lodge is a winter cross country skiing center that had a dining room for guests. We had dinner in the dining

room. After dinner we put on our skis around 10:00 p.m. and skied up the road to Rock Creek Lake, across the lake into the cabin arriving at 12:00 midnight.

That same year on April 1, 1981 Doug Robinson and I skied from Mammoth to the cabin. We skied up over Duck Pass, up over Pika Lake and the next morning climbed down backwards into the McGee Creek Canyon, skied down to Steelhead Lake, crossed over into Pioneer Basin, skied down to Mono Creek, up the creek and over Mono Pass down Mono Pass, into the Bear Creek Spire cirques and down to the cabin.

From 1981 on I used the cabin extensively in the winter to ski in for three or four days. Gary McCain, a Bakersfield friend, was a frequent companion. Many times we were not able to leave Bakersfield until late Friday afternoon. We would drive to Bishop, have dinner, usually some wine and drive up to the east fork and regardless of the time load up our packs and ski to the cabin many times being guided by head lamps. If we arrived early enough at the east fork where we still had light we liked to ski up the "Outhouse" Trail. It was called the Outhouse Trail because the trail started at an outhouse at the Rock Creek Winter Lodge. The trail was quite scenic and basically followed Rock Creek up to the Rock Creek Winter Lodge. There we would say hello to Jan, the proprietor, cross the bridge over Rock Creek and head up the Rock Creek Road to the cabin. In the winter Rock Creek Lake was usually frozen over and the ice very solid so we would save time by skiing across the lake about one mile to the cabin.

If it was late sometimes the moon would be out and the skiing across the lake in the moonlight was quite spectacular. When we would arrive at the cabin we would sometimes have to shovel out the back door so that we could access the interior of the cabin. I can remember many times where we would arrive to find as much as ten feet of snow stacked against the backdoor which would have to be shoveled out before we could get the door open.

Once inside the cabin we would get the potbelly stove burning with almond wood we had hauled in the previous summer from the San Joaquin Valley. Once the stove was roaring it would heat the interior of the cabin to the extent that you could walk around the interior in a short-sleeve shirt even though it could be below freezing outside.

The interior of Rock Creek cabin was rustic. It was basically one room with the west side devoted to cooking and eating and the east side for gathering around the potbelly stove. Once the stove was roaring the cabin was quite comfortable. There was no electricity or phones or T.V. and no running water in the winter. Light was by kerosene lamps. All meals were either by barbeque on an outdoor grill or cooked either on the wood stove or on a propane burner.

In the wintertime we retrieved fresh water from the spring that ran next to the cabin. We would have to break through the ice at times to get to the water which we would dip out and pour into large jugs to carry into the cabin. In the summer the spring ran throughout the summer, and water was piped into the cabin from a small reservoir we had constructed on the creek which was gravity-fed into the cabin by PCV pipe.

The spring was great for keeping wine preserved, even in winter, and cooling beer in the summer.

One winter we forgot to disconnect the water system in the late fall and as the temperatures dropped (it can get 10 to 20 below 0 at the cabin in the winter) the water froze in the sink, backed up and flowed over onto the floor. Because the ice had blocked the door from opening into the cabin we had to prop a ladder up to the second story and climb through the windows in the loft and then down into the cabin. There we had to take an ax and break away the ice from the backdoor so we could get it open. We spent the entire afternoon and the next day with hammers and axes breaking ice up on the floor which was one to two inches thick. After that we always remembered to shut the water off in the late fall before the temperature dropped.

There was no indoor plumbing. We had an outhouse that was a little cold in the winter but serviceable.

In the summer Rock Creek Resort, across the lake, had showers that you could rent. The initial charge was only $1.00, but in recent years the price has increased. The showers, however, did have hot water and one could get clean. When we would take our mountain bikes to the cabin it was an easy ride down the trail, around the lake and over to the lodge to have a nice shower and perhaps a cold beer after.

In the winter we liked to arrive early enough so that we could prepare a hearty meal. We had constructed a fire pit behind the cabin. One of our favorite pasttimes was to construct an igloo-type barrier around the fire pit. We would carve out large chunks of frozen snow blocks and build them into a five foot high igloo - to surround the roaring pit fire.

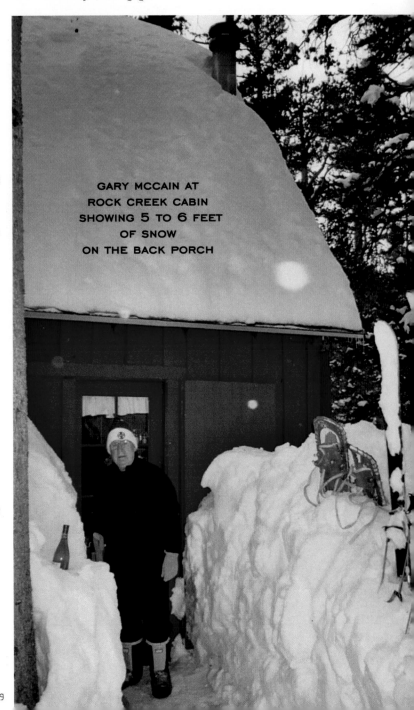

GARY MCCAIN AT
ROCK CREEK CABIN
SHOWING 5 TO 6 FEET
OF SNOW
ON THE BACK PORCH

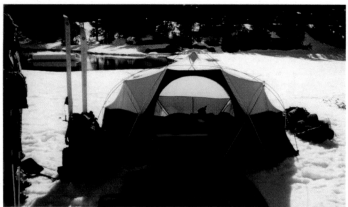

SNOW CAMP AT GEM LAKE AT ABOUT 12,000 FEET

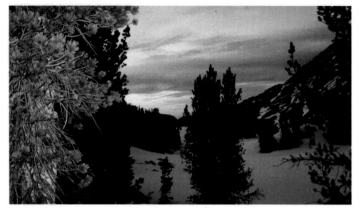

ALPENGLOW LOOKING TO THE EAST OF THE SIERRAS

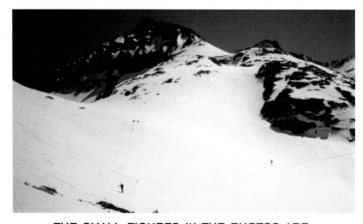

THE SMALL FIGURES IN THE PHOTOS ARE GARY McCAIN AND PAUL RUDDER SKIING BACK TO GEM LAKE FROM THE GIANT BOWLS IN BEAR CREEK SPIRE

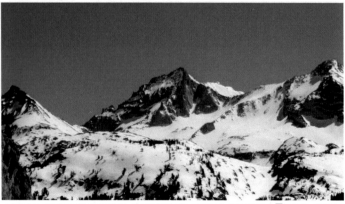

BEAR CREEK SPIRE SHOWING BEAR CREEK PASS AND THE GIANT BOWLS UNDER THE SPIRE

The fire would glaze the interior of the igloo and create a warm interior. We had lawn chairs that we would set in front of the open-pit fire. With a roaring fire and high igloo walls on two sides of the fire pit it was quite warm and comfortable. It was a great place to sit and sip wine and wonder what the rest of the world was doing. We would often sit and sip wine waiting for the fire to burn down so that we could barbeque our steaks. Dinners were usually barbequed steaks, chicken or fish and fresh green salad that we had hauled up in our backpacks with different varieties of pasta. That with some fresh French bread and ample red wine made for a hearty appetizing dinner. At times I remember the temperature being in the single digits or even below zero while we sat in front of the fire sipping our wine without any complaints of cold. Often time snow would fall and the flakes would be illuminated in the fire glow.

Breakfast favorites would be cowboy potatoes and eggs and bacon or pancakes.

On one trip to the cabin in December 1995 we had our usual festive dinner. That night it was a full moon so around midnight Gary McCain and I decided we were going to ski across and around Rock Creek Lake in the full moon. We got out skis on, made our way down to the lake and launched out into the frozen lake. There was a nice frosty, frozen half foot of snow on the lake, and with the full moon it was almost like daylight. The snow was almost corn snow, and we glided easily across the lake in the full moon. We were dressed "full winter" and had no discomfort from the 0 degree temperature. It was an occasion that few other human beings have had an opportunity to experience.

On another occasion I did the same trip with Jerry Dunlap. Jerry felt that it was a very moving experience and for years after would recall skiing across Rock Creek Lake on a full moon.

What Rock Creek cabin did was to provide great access to the Little Lakes basin and the Bear Creek Spire cirque, particularly in the winter.

Many high-country skiers love to make the trip into Bear Creek Spire at 13,000 feet. However, these skiers have to start in the morning at the east fork of Rock Creek with eight or nine miles of travel uphill to Mosquito Flat where the climb begins up through Little Lakes Valley basin. From Mosquito Flat up into the Bear Creek Spire area there is another 2,000 to 3,000 feet of climbing in sparse high altitude oxygen.

It is a long day to ski all the way from the east fork to the high shoulder of Bear Creek Spire to take one run.

Of course the run can be all the way from the shoulder of Bear Creek Spire back down to the east fork. This makes it very difficult to do in one day. Most of the people that want to ski the Bear Creek Spire, pitch winter camp at Treasure Lakes so that they only have a half day climb from Treasure Lakes to where they are going to ski the Bear Creek Spire.

For me having access to Bear Creek Spire, starting at 10,000 feet was a huge advantage.

My favorite trip into the Bear Creek Spire area is to spend the night at the cabin with a tasty dinner, then the next morning after a good hearty breakfast head up the road to Mosquito Flats. From there one can ski up the summer trail buried in snow to Long Lake, which in the winter would be frozen and can be skied across. From there is a climb up another 500 or 600 feet to Gem Lakes, an ideal winter campsite. There is usually open water at Gem Lake which can be filtered for cooking and drinking in the winter. When camped at Gem Lake one can make an early start up the steep far east side of the canyon into the Bear Creek Spire basin. Once up into the basin above the tree line one can pick out various routes to ski the giant bowls. The one I like the best was off of the saddle to the east of Bear Creek Spire. Bear Creek Spire itself at 13,100 feet is not skiable from the top, but one can climb up to the saddle on the east ridge of the mountain to ski the bowls. I have previously skied Bear Creek Spire from almost the top, that is over Bear Creek Spire Pass which is just a few hundred feet from the very top of the mountain.

On one cross country ski trip we accessed Bear Creek Spire Pass by coming up the back side of the spire from Lake Italy. This was on a ski trip from Paiute Pass to Rock Creek Canyon with Gary McCain and Don Williams. The Spire was really not skiable from the top of the pass as it was too steep. We backed down the pass with our skis until we could find a spot to put on the skis and make long traverses. Usually when I camped at Gem Lake we would ski the upper bowls and then when ready return to Gem Lake, climb up to the saddle one more time then ski from there all the way down back to Gem Lake along the eastern canyon which was a fantastic run, particularly if it was corn snow. At Gem Lake we could then have hot tea and soup and later a hot dinner, crawl into our sleeping bags and the next day start the process again.

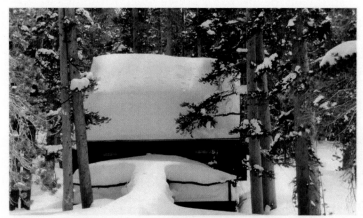
ROCK CREEK CABIN BURIED IN SNOW

In addition to the Bear Creek Spire there were other great areas to ski in the Rock Creek Canyon. One of my favorites was climbing up the canyon behind the cabin to Eastern Brook Lakes, skiing across the two lakes then climbing up the last high ridge before one passed over into Marsh Lake. From that ridge back down through the canyon across both Eastern Brook Lakes and then down the canyon back to the cabin was as good as the skiing can get. The best part was following the canyon from the last Eastern Brook Lake skiing down the whoop-di-dos which were atop the stream and canyon draining east out of Eastern Brook Lakes.

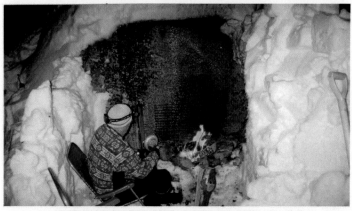
STAYING WARM AND COZY IN OUR IGLOO

Another great ski from the cabin was to climb up the trail to Hilton Lakes just behind Rock Creek Resort and ski down the Hilton Lakes Canyon to Davis Lake - climb up the north side of the canyon and ski down the long canyon into McGee Creek and old Highway 395. One can usually hitch a ride back to Tom's Place for a cold beer and a waiting car.

The cabin was also a delight in the summer. Staying there gave one great access to the beautiful lakes about twenty in number up in the Little Lakes basin.

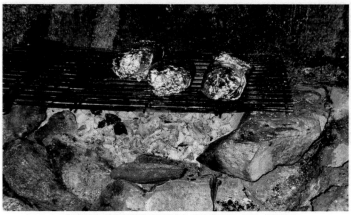
ROCK CREEK CABIN DINNER ON GRILL

The hike to Ruby Lake, a large secluded picturesque lake in a cirque off of Mono Pass trail, was a beautiful destination. Long Lake, Gem Lake and Chicken Foot Lake were other beautiful lakes in the high valley filled with trout with excellent fishing and camping.

One could also go east and hike up to Dorothy and Frances Lakes off the Tamarack Trail. These lakes were very secluded, had few visitors and were a great place for fishing and just relaxing. The canyon up to Tamarack Lake was also a great ski run in the winter.

Another great ski adventure in Rock Creek Canyon was to ski up the Tamarack Trail behind the cabin then take the ridge down Sand Canyon all the way to Swall Meadow. Usually the snow would run out in the spring on the dirt roads above Swall Meadow. It was best to have another vehicle at the snow line to access and come back to Tom's Place for cold beer. The best time to ski Sand Canyon was in the spring with corn snow and short-sleeve weather.

In the summer the Tamarak Trail to the top of Sand Canyon and down the canyon by mountain bike was another favorite journey after the snow had melted out. Again it is best to leave a vehicle at Swall Meadows for the ride back to the cabin or Mammoth.

We always kept a journal at the cabin and all of us recorded our activities as we came and went describing in detail what we did, where we went, what we ate, what we drank and what great fun we had. When arriving at the cabin it was always fun to read the journal and learn what other cabin mates were up to.

In looking back through the journals of the cabin I came across Saturday, August 10, 1991. It would appear on that date that I drove to the cabin in a Ford Aerostar van without four-wheel drive. I had seven people in the vehicle and could not quite make it up the "goat trail" road. Everyone got out and pushed except for me who kept driving. We prayed and got up the hill without a mishap. I had six Soviet Russian friends who had come from the Republic of Moldavia. I had met Alexander Solomonov in the Pamir Mountains in 1987 in Soviet Central Asia where I was climbing Peak Kommunizma and Peak Lenin. We became friendly and before I left I gave him my Timex watch which he admired. He was still wearing it when he came to the U.S.A. We continued to correspond, and I invited them to come to the United States. In 1987 USA and Russia were still in the Cold War, but we were able to get permission for them to come to the USA through our mountain climbing connections. The Russians arrived in New York a week before August 10th and came by Greyhoud Bus to Bakersfield where they stayed at

my house. The Russians were alpinists or mountain climbers. They loved Bakersfield, and the men loved having me take them into the hardware store and the women to the supermarket. They were like kids shopping for candy when visiting these places. The men could not believe the tools and equipment at Home Depot - they had never seen anything like it before. I took the women to Vons and you would have thought they arrived in the promise land. They were amazed in the fresh produce department. They could not believe we had access to such wonderful fruits and vegetables.

Since the men were climbers I thought they would enjoy Rock Creek Canyon, especially the Bear Creek Spire area. They loved the cabin and the mountains.

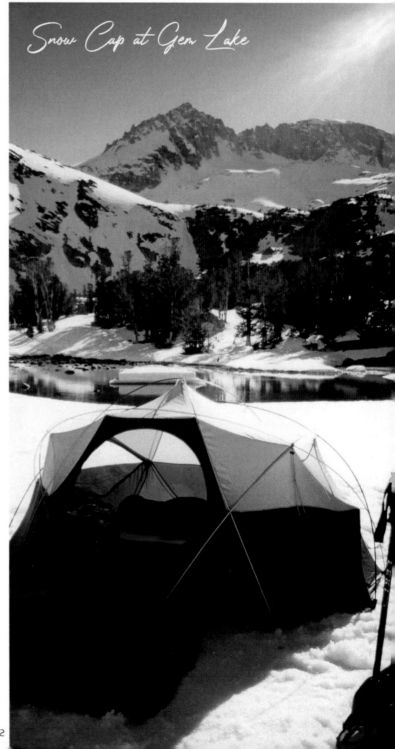

Snow Cap at Gem Lake

We spent the night at the cabin - 08/10/1991 - and the next morning we left early and hiked and climbed our way along the south side of the canyon arriving at Gem Lakes around 1:00 where we had lunch. We then climbed up into the Bear Creek basin area and had a great time taking in the scenery. We did not get back to the cabin until 8:30. We prepared a grand meal - barbequed tri-tip-and we opened several bottles of Cabernet Sauvignon. The conversation was fractured English with a very few words of Russian (Tim). We covered a wide range of topics especially the chaotic situation in the Russian Republics which was unpredictable in the fall of 1991. The conversation was animated and lively. The Russians were used to mountain living since they were all mountaineers and were great guests all sharing the work at the cabin.

The guests:
Alexander (Shasha) and his wife Irina Solomonov; Shasha and Galina Bartchok; Orleg and Raisa Timfenencko

Galina wrote a nice letter in our journal in Russian ending with: "Dasvidaniya Tim," which means goodbye in Russian.

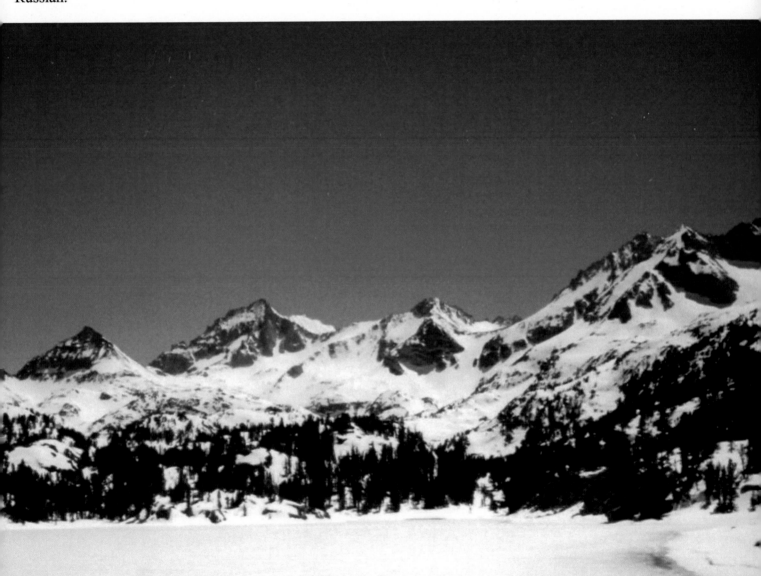

WINTER VIEW OF THE
BEAR CREEK SPIRE
CIRQUE FROM
MARSH LAKE IN
LITTLE LAKES CANYON

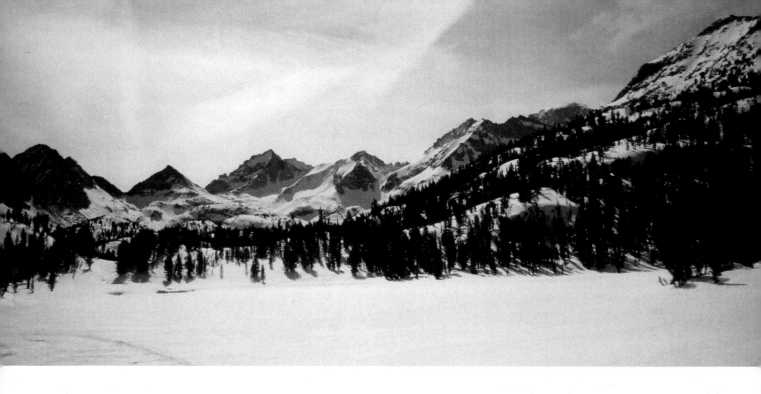

Over the years with the cabin we had many exciting and wonderful experiences. Gary McCain did a lot of work in re-building the sink and cabinets in the kitchen. We had a gang of tri-athletes spend four days at the cabin with Bob Love putting a new roof on the cabin, eating hearty and drinking a few beers. Gary McCain and I became accomplished wood splitters and kept the cabin supplied with our hard-split wood.

One of my favorite things to do at the cabin is to just sit on the front porch on an early cool summer morning with a hot cup of coffee and watch the chipmunks and savor the high altitude environment.

The cabin has been a wonderful experience for my succession of dogs: Penny, Peaches; Blondie, Blossom; Roxy; Rosie; Lulu; and now Susie. They all had great fun coming to the cabin, swimming in the lake, running through the streams, going for hikes and chasing squirrels and chipmunks.

On cold winter nights I would put a pad down by the potbelly stove and have a two or three dog night with my fur friends.

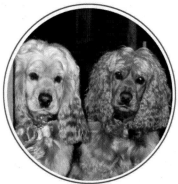

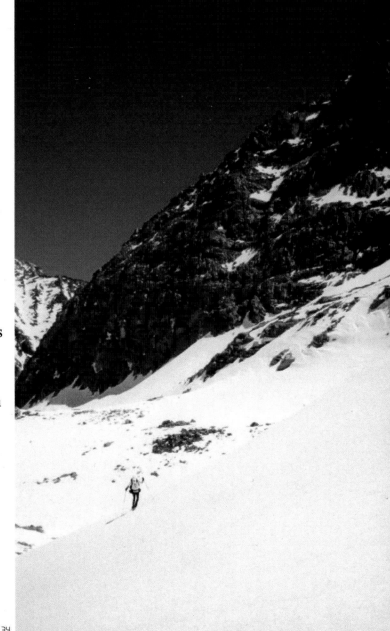

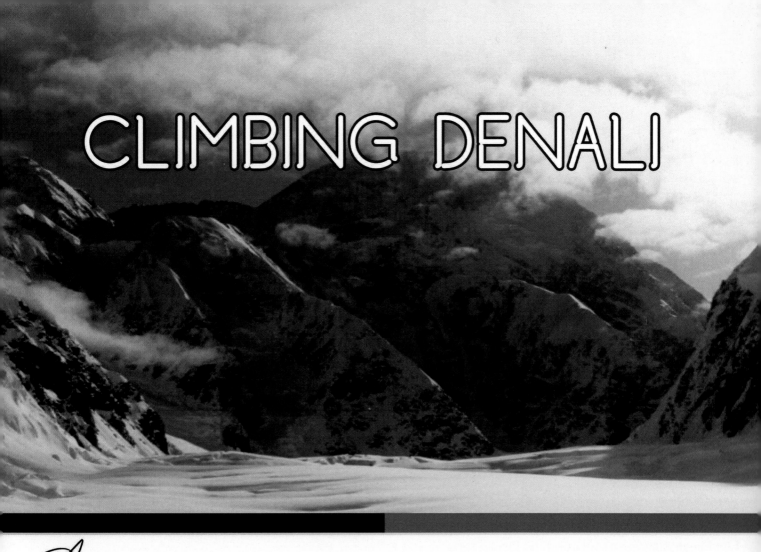

CLIMBING DENALI

At age forty-nine I successfully climbed with a group of ten other climbers to the top of Mt. Denali in Alaska reaching the summit on June 23, 1986. Before 1975 Denali was recognized on maps as Mt. McKinley - named after the American president. However, the mountain has always been known by Alaskans as Denali, a Koyukon Indian name meaning "the great one." In 1975 the Alaska legislature asked the U.S. Federal Government to officially change the name of the mountain from Mt. McKinley to Denali as all previous attempts to do so were blocked by members of the congressional delegation from Ohio, the home state of President William McKinley who served as president from 1837 until his assassination in 1901. My climbing companions, knowing that I was a triathlete and had competed in Hawaii's Ironman Triathlon, asked me to compare the climb of Denali to competing in Hawaii's Ironman. I consider these two adventures to be athletic ultra-endurance events and they can in fact be compared in one significant manner - it is not the distance of the Ironman at 140 miles or the height (Denali) at 20,320 feet but the conditions under which each event is performed that make both of the them so incredibly tough.

As Ironman competitors who have endured the 2.4 mile open-ocean swim, the 112 mile bike race and the 26.2 mile marathon run can attest, it is the ocean swell and chops in the swim, the unrelenting headwinds in the bike race and the blistering heat and humidity in the run (marathon) rather than the distance itself of 140 miles that constitutes the real challenge. If you can persevere through the conditions you can do the distance.

Alaska's Denali at 20,370 feet is not the highest in the world; yet it has the most severe and unpredictable weather of any of the world's major summits. Its peak is 36 degrees latitude further north than Mt. Everest and less than 200 miles south of the arctic circle. It lies in the direct path of the Siberian Gulf of Alaska storm creation center and at its height of 20,370 feet receives the full blast at its upper elevations of the jet stream.

According to the Denali National Park Reserve Weather Service, the temperature on Denali during the summer climbing season can average -40Fahrenheit accompanied by winds of eighty to one hundred miles per hour lasting for several days.

With the right set of climate and weather circumstances the temperature can plummet to 80 degrees below 0 - which it did on our climb. The combined effect of the cold, wind and altitude makes the upper regions of the mountain one of the most hostile climates on earth.

Another condition Denali climbers must contend with is high altitude sickness (HAS) - headache, loss of appetite, irritability, weakness, nausea and disturbed breathing and sleep which are all common results of climbing at altitude. There is no way of predicting who will or will not develop altitude illness, and no medicine is a proven preventative.

The idea to climb Denali first occurred to me in June of 1984 when I was a tourist in Alaska. I had taken the train from Anchorage to Fairbanks and made a stop at Denali National Park to take the bus ride to Wonder Lake to see Mt. Denali. Upon the return to the McKinley Lodge a group of Denali climbers were returning from their climb from the mountain. I was extremely curious and peppered them with questions about the climb, their equipment, food, health, et cetera. They probably found me a nosy pest; yet I formed the idea,

"I can do this."

I had been thinking about climbing Denali for a couple of years. I wrote to the Denali National Park Service for information. In the brochure that they sent me describing the hazards of a Denali climb, the parks people who keep records of each ascent set out the requirements of a successful climbing party:

Each member must posses superior mountaineering skills, stamina, conditioning, equipment and the ability to survive in severe arctic conditions.

Experience has shown that even these qualifications do not guarantee safety or success.

I was at that time a forty-nine year old age-group triathlete.

Was I up to this challenge?

The pre-conditioning program was a snap. By this time I had completed three Hawaii Ironman Championships finishing 4th place in the 40-50 age group. I knew I could make the physical and mental conditioning. In the four months before the climb I kept up my triathlete training program - 10 miles per week in the pool; 150 miles per week on the bicycle; 40 miles per week running on the roads. As tune-up I competed in the Los Angeles Triathlon Championship series at Bonelli Park (first place master for the series); the Bakersfield Bud Light triathlon (first place); Phoenix United States Triathlon series race (first place in the age forty-five to forty-nine).

Aerobically and mentally I was ready to climb. However, the training in the warm, dry southern California weather did not prepare one to carry loads of sixty to eighty pounds for prolonged hours in severe cold weather.

Also I had no real track record as a mountain climber. I had climbed Mt. Orizaba in Mexico (18,496 feet); other Mexican volcanoes: Popocatepetl (17,800 feet), Popocatepetl's next door neighbor, Itzaccihuatl (17,334 feet). I had also climbed in the Sierra Nevadas: five times to the top of Mt. Whitney (14,500 feet) and some other lesser peaks. I did have extensive high altitude ski mountaineering experience in the Sierra Nevada mountains.

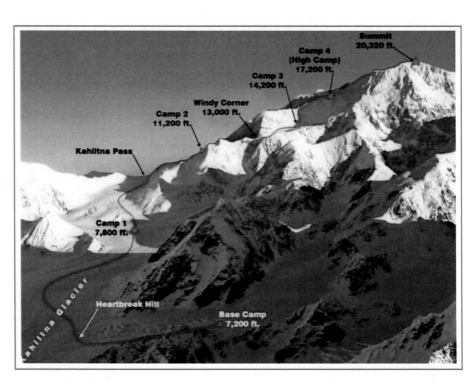

Summit 20,320 ft.

Camp 4 (High Camp) 17,200 ft.

Camp 3 14,200 ft.

Windy Corner 13,000 ft.

Camp 2 11,200 ft.

Kahiltna Pass

Camp 1 7,800 ft.

Kahiltna Glacier

Heartbreak Hill

Base Camp 7,200 ft.

I would be climbing with experienced climbers. Climbers are an elite group of athletes with highly developed physical, technical and aerobic skills and abilities. Could I stay up with these people? In climbing Denali was I in way over my head?

As a neophyte climber with limited technical skills I was "untested" and an "unknown quantity" to my veteran Alaskan guide, Gary Bocarde. I met Bocarde, an experienced Denali mountain guide, in Anchorage in early June for an equipment checking session with the other ten men and one woman, members of our climbing group, for an orientation conference. Conversation ranged over the technical equipment we had assembled. I can talk bike parts, wetsuits or running gear but I was out of my element discussing climbing equipment: ascenders, harnesses, crampons, belays.

Bocarde asked to inspect my ascender.

"What's that?" I asked. Gary gave me a startled look and said, "That's what's going to get you out of the ice crevasse you may fall into...you better learn how to use it and use it well..."

Later, on the trip, after we landed by ski plane on the Kahiltna glacier I saw my first real crevasse. A crevasse is a deep crack that forms in a glacier. The Kahiltna glacier is several hundred feet deep and many miles long. When you have your first look into one of those crevasses and do not see a bottom...you just see blue getting bluer and bluer and then black, it strikes terror in your heart.

After looking into the crevasse I learned quickly how to use the ascender, the climbing harness and the shoulder sling - the equipment that would prevent us from dangling upside down in the crevasse. Fear motivates rapid learning.

Bocarde, the owner guide of Mountain Trip, had been guiding for thirteen years and had fourteen successful summits on Denali, many over technically difficult routes. He had climbing credits in China, Russia and the Himalayas. Susan Havens, Bocarde's wife and co-guide, was also an experienced mountaineer with impressive climbing credits including the first successful woman's climb of Ama Dablam in Napal.

We were to conduct our climb in early June. The snow conditions and weather are usually best during that time. Later in the summer the lower glaciers, such as the Kahiltna and the Muldrow upon which we would be spending a good deal of our time, become a problem with melting snow bridges over crevasses and more severe weather and heavier snowfall.

Bocarde outlined our climb plan - we were to fly our climbers and equipment by ski plane from Talkeetna,

Alaska, a small Alaskan village at the south base of the mountian into the base camp on the Kahiltna glacier at 7,000 feet. The Kahiltna Glacier is thirty-five miles long and several hundred feet deep. From there we would double-carry our equipment expedition-style to establish a series of seven to eight camps on the glacier on the west side of the mountain. We would then attempt to establish a camp at 18,000 feet to launch a summit attempt depending upon the weather and the strength and condition of the climbers. If we made the summit we would descend down the north side of the mountain to the Harper glacier, the spectacular Karsten's ridge, connecting into the giant Muldrow glacier. We would follow the glacier which is forty miles long to its base and cross the historic McGonagal pass where we would leave the ice and traverse 20 miles over tundra hills and glacial streams to Wonder Lake in Denali National Park. From there we would take the park bus to the Denali park headquarters and catch the Alaska Railroad back to Anchorage.

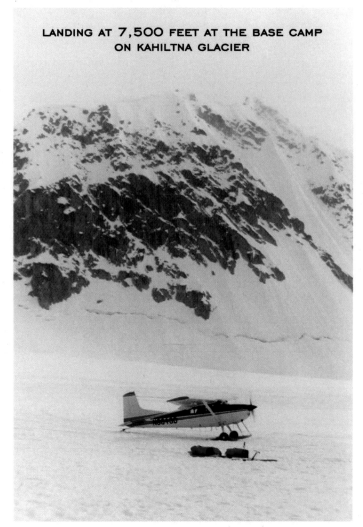

LANDING AT 7,500 FEET AT THE BASE CAMP ON KAHILTNA GLACIER

The climbing-hiking portion of our trip would include ascending from 7,000 feet to the summit of Denali at 20,300 feet and then descending over 18,000 feet to Wonder Lake, a distance of over 140 miles. Our trip was expected to last twenty-one to thirty days subject to weather and physical conditioning.

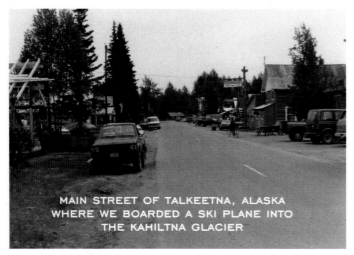

MAIN STREET OF TALKEETNA, ALASKA
WHERE WE BOARDED A SKI PLANE INTO
THE KAHILTNA GLACIER

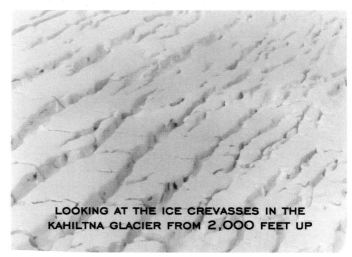

LOOKING AT THE ICE CREVASSES IN THE
KAHILTNA GLACIER FROM 2,000 FEET UP

From 7,000 feet there was usually always fresh snow as it snowed almost every day, if only a few inches. The initial climb from 7,000 to 14,000 feet was on snow shoes. From 14,000 feet on climbing was always with crampons.

The initial climb from 7,000 feet to 14,000 feet was plain drudgery. Each climber was responsible for 150 pounds of personal gear, food, fuel and climbing equipment. On Denali there were no mules, llamas or sherpas. Everything was people-carried. Each section of our initial climb up the Kahiltna glacier was covered twice - carry up one half of your one hundred and fifty pound load, dig out a camp, protect it from the wind. Bury all of the load in the snow (to protect against the scavenger ravens), descend down to 7,000 feet, and return with the other one half of your load the next day. Exposed equipment, backpacks, food bags and other gear could be ripped apart by the scavenger ravens if not buried in the snow.

On the initial first phase of each morning climb each person carried a backpack with sixty to seventy pounds of equipment, fuel and food and in addition pulled a sled harnessed to the waist with another seventy or more pounds making up the one hundred and fifty pounds each person was responsible for. Fortunately, the loads lessened quickly as we used up the fuel and food in ascending the glacier.

The twelve members of our party were on four ropes - three to a rope for safety. With 50 feet apart there was no conversation during the climb, and the wind which was usually always present made it almost impossible to even shout communication to the climber in front or behind. The first part of the trip was very lonely.

Some days were spent "nailed" in the tent by severe weather, particularly fierce winds.

Each climber wore a climbing harness snapped onto the rope by an ascender and carabiner and was warned never to un-hook - only at camp, and only after the guides had stomped the area for crevasses and snow bridges.

The park service issued this warning:

"All climbers should be roped for any glacier travel and must be familiar with crevasse rescue techniques. Several climbers have died from un-roped falls on the mountain. Before un-roping, the camp area should be thoroughly checked for possible crevasses."

The reason was that high winds often blew snow across crevasse openings creating weak snow bridges that could easily collapse under weight.

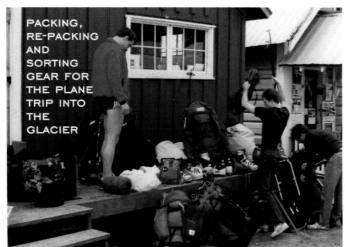

PACKING, RE-PACKING AND SORTING GEAR FOR THE PLANE TRIP INTO THE GLACIER

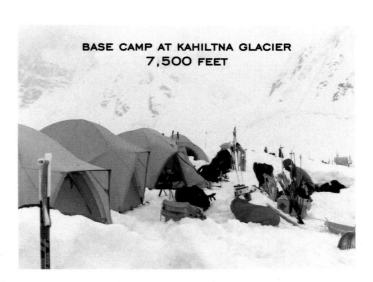

BASE CAMP AT KAHILTNA GLACIER
7,500 FEET

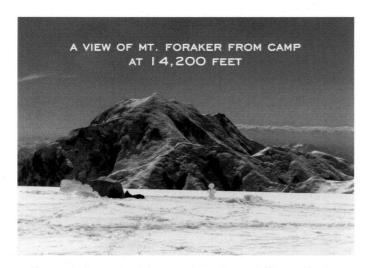

A VIEW OF MT. FORAKER FROM CAMP AT 14,200 FEET

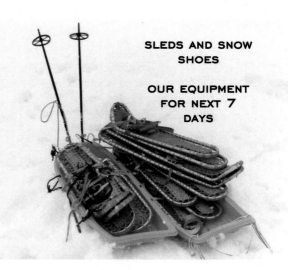

SLEDS AND SNOW SHOES

OUR EQUIPMENT FOR NEXT 7 DAYS

The week-long double carry up the Kahiltna glacier was pure drudgery, but it did serve a strategic purpose - it allowed us to acclimate gradually and avoid the dreaded high altitude sickness (HAS). We also lightened our loads of fuel and food.

The mountain is cruel. At 14,000 we witnessed the evacuation of two young Swiss climbers by rescue rangers. The pair had died in their tent from carbon monoxide asphyxiation from the fumes of a non-ventilated stove during a storm. When we saw them being rescued they were frozen stiff like human popsicles as they had been dead for a few days before we discovered them.

After 14,000 feet, in addition to the drudgery of double carrying, there was frequent exposure to real danger. We had to ascend a 2,000 foot "headwall" on the West Buttress on fixed ropes with ice axes and crampons in gale force winds with our seventy pound backpacks. A slip could send one cascading on hard ice thousands of feet below. Even though the lower slopes were not usually more than 30 to 50 degrees, slips could be disastrous and carry a climber hundreds of feet on ice or hard-pack if he was not able to self-arrest. Most climbers who fell on 30 degree slopes would accelerate without being able to self-arrest and end up smashing into rocks or being catapulted over a cliff. Rescue could be extremely hazardous or even non-existent.

At 16,000 feet we were exhausted and ready to camp only to find an exposed mountain shoulder, hard, icy, wind-blown and uninviting. This was a planned stop, and for a few minutes we explored and considered bivouacking in ice caves dug by earlier climbers but found them small, cold and dark. Some of us experienced claustrophobia in the caves, and all agreed that even though it was extremely cold and with high-fierce winds it would less miserable to continue climbing.

On the way to the 16,000 foot camp we could see the famous Japanese Couloir - where four members of a Japanese climbing team were caught in a fierce storm and trapped on their rope against an icy cliff. They froze to death in place and in 1986 still remained there on their climbing rope. Apparently it was thought too dangerous to try to retrieve their bodies; as far as I know are still there. It was a chilling sight. A couloir is a narrow chute.

The next possible camp was at 17,000 feet, and the climb there took us up along an icy ridge in blasting winds bordered on each side by icy cliffs. As we inched up through the hard ice packed between granite outcroppings I thought of the prospect of having to double-climb the same route yet again the next day with the same back breaking pack - UGH!

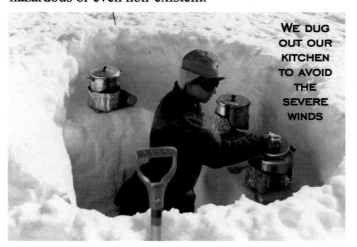

WE DUG OUT OUR KITCHEN TO AVOID THE SEVERE WINDS

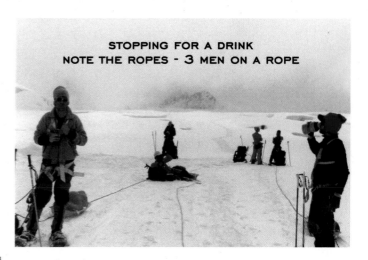

STOPPING FOR A DRINK
NOTE THE ROPES - 3 MEN ON A ROPE

At 17,000 feet we pitched camp in an igloo-style barricaded pocket dug by previous climbers. At this elevation we were now in the perpetual deep freeze zone. Here, except for what was swept away by the winds, nothing ever melts or disintegrates. Footprints, trash and human waste remain "forever" frozen and preserved in the sub-freezing climate.

At this altitude frostbite becomes an ever-present danger. Metal objects such as an ice ax or tent stake would freeze and stick immediately to exposed flesh. Almost everything that you did not keep in your sleeping bag would freeze including toothpaste and contact lens solution.

The altitude was now a challenge and affected every climber to some degree. Breathing became laborious; headache and nausea accompanied exertions; appetite diminished; patience and tempers were short.

Irritability can easily spring up between close friends and climbing partners during a stay at high altitude. A nagging fear, doubt, or feeling of guilt can easily grow in one's mind and prove mentally exhausting as well as potentially dangerous. Personality change may bring out latent domineering tendencies in anyone and can be extremely upsetting in a group relationship. Being on the mountain may precipitate a variety of phobias, including claustrophobia from living in close quarters, which can lead to panic with an overwhelming desire to run away. In some extreme cases a single climber has been known to leave the group in an attempt to descend by himself which can lead to fatal consequences. Judgment can be affected.

We read in the brochure put out by the Denali Park Service that many high altitude climbing accidents may be attributed to such lack of judgement. It is important that climbers realize in advance that their mental functions will be impaired. Planning should be thorough and complete to avoid a critical situation which poor judgement and slow thinking would magnify. For example, sudden impulsive decisions to go on or to return must be considered carefully.

Joseph Wilcox, a climbing leader in a 1967 McKinley party, wrote in his diary:

"With five people crammed in the tent, morale decreased rapidly. There was no interest in cooking meals and by the next day no one was even interested in melting drinking water. We found ourselves very apathetic - not caring whether or not we got enough to drink or eat or if our gear was wet - we just lay there and waited with little or no sleep ... by morning the cold had taken its toll. One climber had numb feet and another, numb fingers...

We had been warned to expect these changes in our temperament, and we worked together to minimize their effect on group morale.

After 17,000 feet the next move was an exhausting steep climb to 18,000 feet on a fixed rope with wracked and ice axes to an area called Denali Pass, a wind-racked ice saddle between the north peak of Denali at 19,000 feet and the "true summit" of the south peak at 20,300 feet. Here the wind rules, and for two and a half days we remained "nailed" in our tents by the fierce wind and -60 degree temperature. We only ventured outside our tents and sleeping bags for absolute necessity using the privy and gathering in the guide tent for meals. The hours passed slowly and miserably.

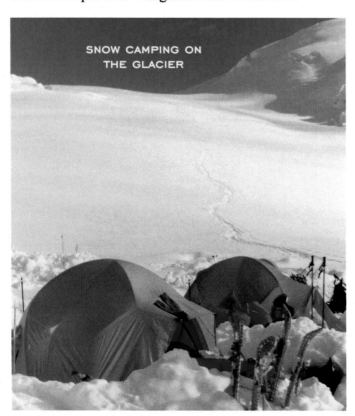

SNOW CAMPING ON
THE GLACIER

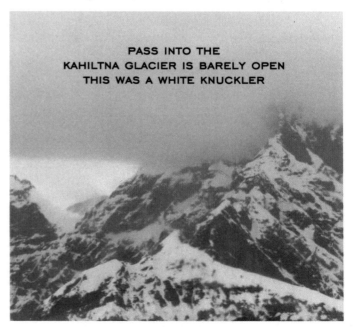

PASS INTO THE
KAHILTNA GLACIER IS BARELY OPEN
THIS WAS A WHITE KNUCKLER

A major hazard of a Mt. McKinley climb is frostbite and hypothermia. McKinley presents a combination of long exposure, severe weather, high altitude, low temperature and low humidity which makes it one of the most severe climates on earth. Mountaineering literature contains numerous vivid accounts of frostbite on Mt. McKinley such as Bradford Wasburn's article that appeared in the American Alpine Club journal. During the 1976 climbing season there were fifty-three reported cases of frostbite; fourteen of these required medical attention. Three 1967 McKinley climbers had their feet frostbitten while they were in their sleeping bags primarily because they had little to eat and were dehydrated. Subsequently, two of these climbers lost portions of their toes. These climbers were at 18,000 feet (Denali Pass) for six days with temperatures of -50 and -60 degrees Fahrenheit in winds of ninety to one hundred miles per hour. Doug Scott, a McKinley guide who was involved in the rescue of these climbers from Denali Pass, wrote in his diary:

"As we made our way slowly down we were surprised to see figures ahead. We could make out two climbers sitting in the snow with equipment strewn all around them ... they were two lads of about twenty. One was wearing a black silk glove that had been ripped apart to reveal yellowing fingers, frozen solid; the other was just sitting stupefied in the snow, his head bowed over his own useless, frozen hands. Yellow fingers was quite chirpy; joking at the coincidence of our meeting at the pass like this. My friend asked why his hands were exposed and he received a confident flip reply. We told him that he had frostbite, and that he would probably lose his fingers, and maybe his entire hand. 'What do you mean frostbite?' asked yellow fingers. We patiently explained, got his gloves and other clothes out of his sack and did what we could to make them both warmer. We heard later that the two lads had to face extensive amputation of fingers, toes, hands and feet despite the treatment available at the Anchorage Hospital."

Body tissue which is frozen, thawed and re-frozen will be damaged much more than tissue which is frozen only once.

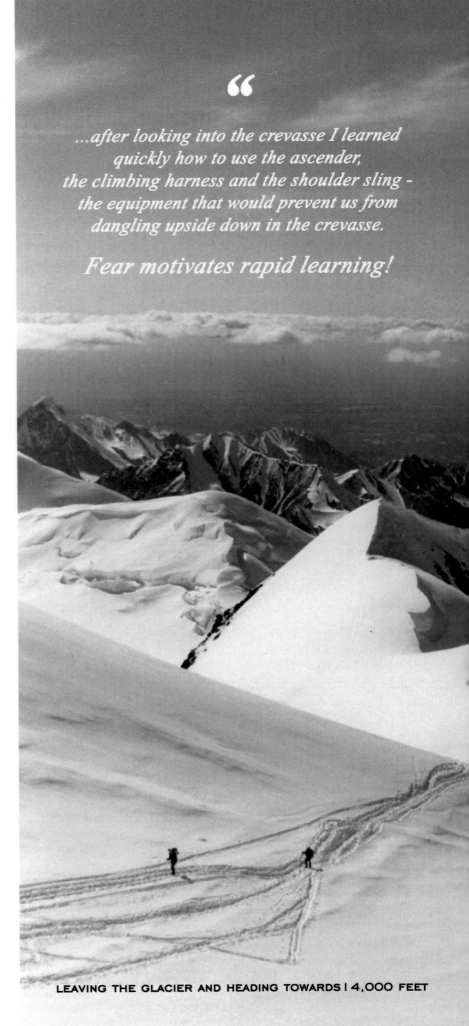

"

...after looking into the crevasse I learned quickly how to use the ascender, the climbing harness and the shoulder sling - the equipment that would prevent us from dangling upside down in the crevasse.

Fear motivates rapid learning!

LEAVING THE GLACIER AND HEADING TOWARDS 14,000 FEET

Two Korean climbers, acutely ill and delirious from high altitude sickness, were brought to our camp at 18,000 feet by exhausted rescuers and bivouacked with us for thirty hours before the weather permitted further descent. One climber was delirious from high altitude edema, either lung or brain, and spent the time waiting for rescue mumbling unintelligibly.

The Kahiltna Denali Rescue Operations could not get a helicopter to 18,000 feet but were able to land at 17,000 feet. The problem was to get the semi-unconscious Korean from 18,000 feet to 17,000 feet so that he could be rescued. His companion had revived somewhat with liquids, hot tea and coffee and would be able to descend the 1,000 feet roped to a rescuer. The unconscious Korean was placed in a sleeping bag with all of his belongings. The bag was then wrapped in rope like a mummy. Fortunately the rescuers had brought rope with them, and we were all able to lower the unconscious Korean in his sleeping bag down a 1,000 feet chute to the 17,000 feet level where the helicopter was able to fly him back to Talkeetna. After the climb was over we heard that the Koreans were taken to the hospital in Anchorage and had made a good recovery.

One must really admire the helicopter pilots that attempt to rescue injured or stranded climbers at high altitude. One pilot, Russ Hunter, with a great deal of helicopter experience on McKinley stated:

"Landing a Chinook helicopter on McKinley is like driving a car into a garage at forty miles per hour and trying to stop before you hit the back wall."

As part of the warnings that the park service issues to climbers they are told that helicopter assistance is not always possible because of severe weather. The first thing that a party should do is try to get an injured or ill climber to a lower elevation where they could possibly be evacuated by fixed-wing aircraft. All climbing groups confronted with an emergency situation should first consider what they can do to handle the situation on the their own. Next they should try to enlist the help of other climbers in the area, and finally only when all other options have been tried should they request additional assistance.

By this time the wind and the cold and the physical exhaustion in helping rescue the Koreans had depleted our physical and mental resources and an abandonment of the summit attempt appeared imminent. Gary Bocarde felt that it would be suicidal to try for the top in the wind and cold. I understood why only about twenty percent of the groups who try to climb Denali make the summit. We were physically capable but weather conditions were horrible.

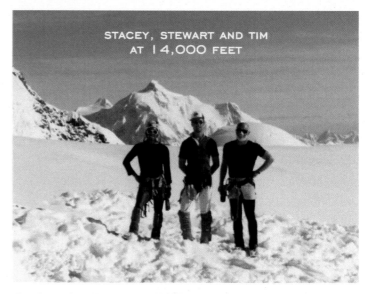

STACEY, STEWART AND TIM AT 14,000 FEET

On June 23rd, as we talked about breaking camp to head down the mountain, the wind suddenly died. While still bitter cold, the conditions outside the tent were tolerable. You could stand up without being blown over by the wind. Gary said, "Let's go to the summit."

From 18,000 to 20,000 feet the climb was fairly routine trekking up 35 to 45 degree ice slopes on rope. Although covered by broken misty clouds the last five hundred feet to the summit presented some spectacular views of the mountain's grandeur.

The trail to the summit wound along the top of an icy cornice bordered on one side by shear vertical drops and icy overhangs of thousands of feet.

When we reached the summit on June 23, 1986 at 4:00 p.m. it was an almost balmy -5 degrees with misty clouds and a light breeze. All of us in the party who made the summit attribute it to Gary Bocarde's craft. After photos and many high-fives the return down the mountain to the Denali Pass at 18,000 feet was uneventful.

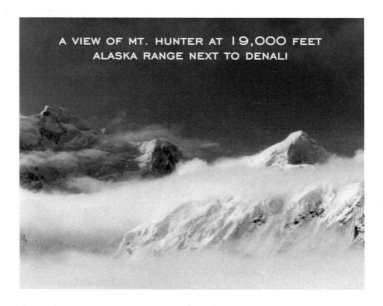

A VIEW OF MT. HUNTER AT 19,000 FEET ALASKA RANGE NEXT TO DENALI

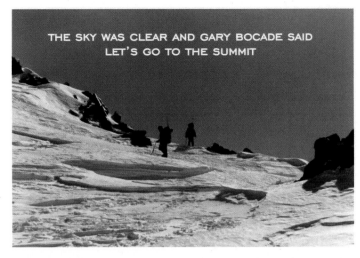

THE SKY WAS CLEAR AND GARY BOCADE SAID
LET'S GO TO THE SUMMIT

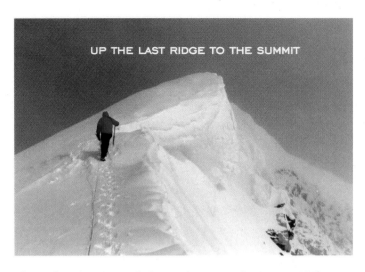

UP THE LAST RIDGE TO THE SUMMIT

Even though it was late in the day, in Alaska in June it would be light past midnight. We had come up the south side of the mountain, and now we were going to descend on the north side to Denali National Park.

Those in our party who thought the descent of the mountain down the north side to Wonder Lake would be anticlimactic were in for a shocker!

Later I likened our descent of the mountain to the continuous and unexpected perils encountered by Indiana Jones, in the movie "Raiders of the Lost Ark." Everywhere we encountered a multiplicity of ways one could kill himself!

Descending the Muldrow Glacier with its awesome ice falls, and down the precipitous icy spine of Karsten's Ridge my senses were buffeted - hours of back-breaking drudgery hauling our heavy packs broken by stretches of adrenalin- charged stark fear from the dizzying heights, tempered by the spectacular otherworldly beauty of the Alaska range.

At the Harper Ice Fall there were giant ice blocks hundreds of feet tall that had fallen off the mountain down onto the glacier. There were moaning glaciers; ice crevasses hundreds of feet deep; ice pools; rotten snow bridges - all of which were part of nature's

obstacles that impeded our descent. It was as if the mountain was telling us, "You made the summit, but see if you are strong enough to get down." Every day we could see and hear avalanches cascading down onto the glacier.

The descent down the Karsten's Ridge still sticks in my mind and causes a chill down my spine when I recall it. The ridge is very narrow, only about two feet wide and steep. Again we are three on a rope. Now we have backpacks loaded with gear including the snow shoes and sleds we used to haul everything to Denali Pass. We took each down step with crampons one at a time on ice buried in a foot of snow, our sleds on the top of the packs buffeted by the winds. To our immediate right is a cliff with a drop - 1,000 feet. The temperature is now -35 degrees, and even with my winter climbing gear I am sweating like on a mid-summer day. The intense concentration on getting each down step in place and securing the ice axe became physically and mentally exhausting after hundreds of feet of descent.

At last we reached the end of the enormous Muldrow Glacier. We clamored over slick black ice covered with sand to reach firm earth on the other side of the glacial moraine.

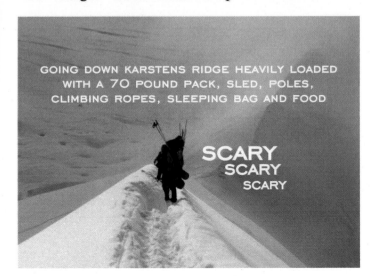

GOING DOWN KARSTENS RIDGE HEAVILY LOADED
WITH A 70 POUND PACK, SLED, POLES,
CLIMBING ROPES, SLEEPING BAG AND FOOD

SCARY
SCARY
SCARY

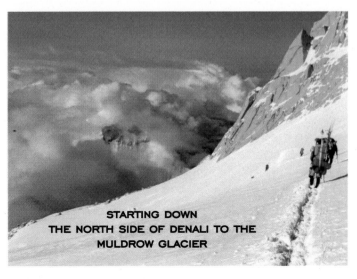

STARTING DOWN
THE NORTH SIDE OF DENALI TO THE
MULDROW GLACIER

We were now on a dirt trail leaving the glacier. The dirt and green scrub emitted a sensuous welcome aroma after eighteen days on the snow and ice. A clump of brilliant purple alpine flowers was a visual treat. We moved lightly with our heavy loads up and over the historic McGonagall Pass to gaze out on the great tundra plain below, leading some forty miles in the distance to Wonder Lake, our destination.

The momentary feeling of joy that the worst was over soon disappeared. Like before, as we descended again down the steep McGonagall Pass still packed with snow, several of us crashed through rotten snow bridges into the icy creek several feet underneath.

We were still carrying fifty plus pound packs loaded with equipment and climbing gear and wearing heavy climbing boots and extreme weather clothing. We were poorly equipped to walk through mud, tundra bogs and glacial stream-crossings over the next thirty-five miles.

Those of us who had carried mosquito netting over the summit had some temporary relief from the swarms of bugs that plagued us in the boggy tundra.

Although slogging through the tundra and bogs was miserable the unusually clear warm weather and the night-less Alaskan summer combined to present us with some awesome vistas of the Alaska range and its crown jewel, Denali.

Only ten miles from Wonder Lake, our destination, one last great obstacle remained - to cross the mile-wide McKinley River. This was a glacier-fed stream whose depth can vary five feet or more per hour depending on the amount of, rain and melt-off from the Muldrow Glacier. The river could be crossed at low water only about two hours a day. We had to time the low water point between the previous day's run off and the new day's melt.

We picked our way up and down the river bank for miles looking for stretches in the swift ice water that would not be more than waist high. Water any higher would grab heavy packs and submerge the hiker in the swift icy current which could be extremely dangerous. By forming human chains in waist-deep water - all roped - we forged across but not before two of our party were swept into the current and lost some gear. Fortunately they recovered with the only injury being submerged in icy cold water. By the time we successfully crossed the river we and our equipment were all wet from the icy water.

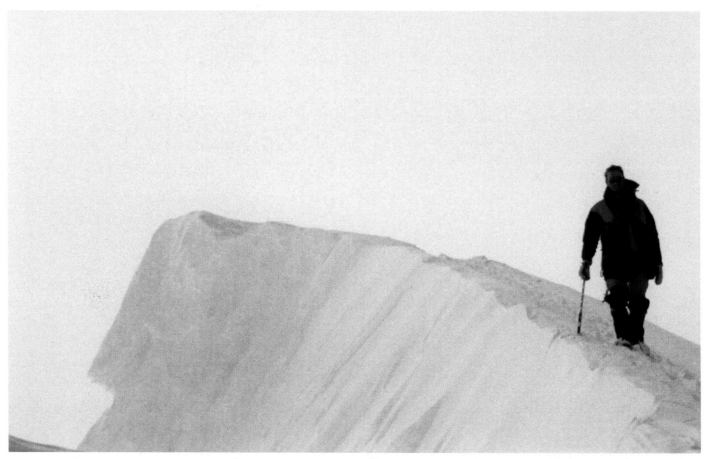

After crossing the McKinley River only a few miles remained, but typical of Alaska these miles were lined with deep tundra bogs that filled our heavy hiking boots with soggy mud and stirred up clouds of mosquitos to bite exposed flesh.

At last, Wonder Lake! One hundred and forty miles! Twelve exhausted climbers un-bathed and un-shaven for four weeks stumbled aboard a Denali Park tour bus of gawking squeaky-clean tourists in their clean outdoor mountain finery. Most of the tourists looked as if they had just posed for a Patagonia outback catalog.

After the initial shock of seeing these mud-spattered creatures the tourists were asking questions and sharing their lunches with us. The bus ride of thirty-five miles brought us to Denali National Park. Before catching the train to Anchorage we descended on a salmon fry - a smorgasbord outdoor cook-out where you could eat all you wanted for $5.00. The owner did not know what hit him as twelve starved climbers ate just about everything he had on the premises. Stuffed and content we then caught the Alaskan Railroad for the train ride back to Anchorage and the end of the trip. Even though the scenery was magnificent on the train most of us fell asleep.

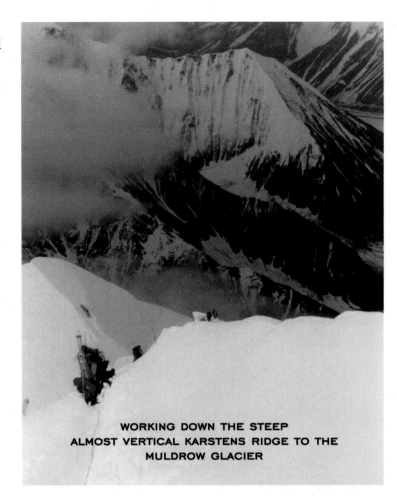

WORKING DOWN THE STEEP ALMOST VERTICAL KARSTENS RIDGE TO THE MULDROW GLACIER

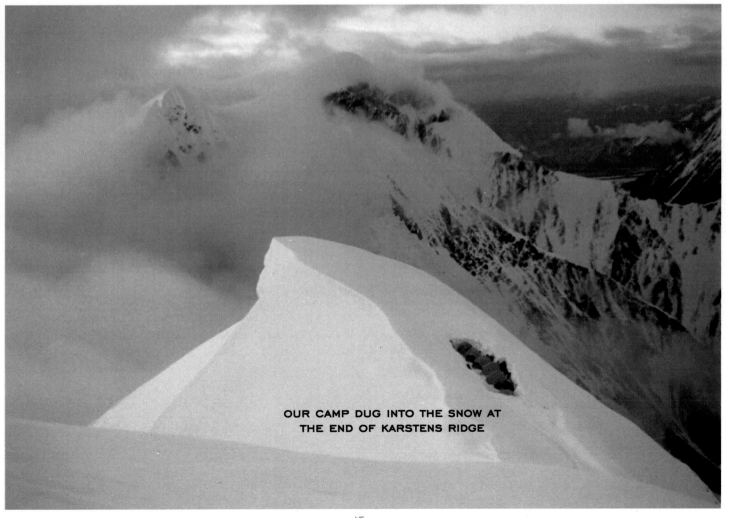

OUR CAMP DUG INTO THE SNOW AT THE END OF KARSTENS RIDGE

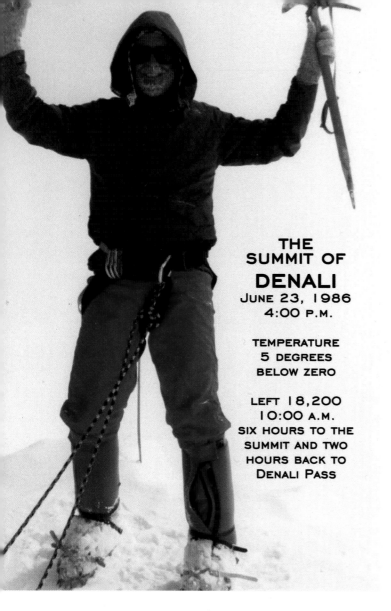

**THE
SUMMIT OF
DENALI**
JUNE 23, 1986
4:00 P.M.

TEMPERATURE
5 DEGREES
BELOW ZERO

LEFT 18,200
10:00 A.M.
SIX HOURS TO THE
SUMMIT AND TWO
HOURS BACK TO
DENALI PASS

My truthful assessment of the trip:
Eighty percent drudgery,
fifteen percent stark terror and
five percent joy.

In excellent physical condition, even before the
start of the trip, at one hundred and seventy pounds
I was now down to a "hard as nails" one hundred
and sixty pounds with a BMI of ten percent and
probably in the best cardiovascular condition of my
life. I would have to say again that one strong
lesson I took from that experience was that on
Denali there are an awful lot of ways for a person
to kill himself.

However as time went by and the stark terror experiences faded I was more taken by the description
of Alfred Hulse Brooks, an early Alaska explorer
from 1865 -1900 who wrote about Denali:

"Were the day clear I could see Mt. McKinley from
the window...I picture in my mind its stupendous
height...many have assailed its flanks; some have
proclaimed untruths about it; some have climbed
by great effort well up the slopes; a very few, the
best by natural selection, have reached the summit
and attained the broad vision denied those at lower
altitudes."

Denali was first climbed by Hudson Struck, a
British native who became the episcopal archdea-
con of the Yukon. He wrote a wonderful book
about his journey and experiences as an episcopal
missionary in the Yukon: 1,000 Miles by Dogsled -
fascinating reading.

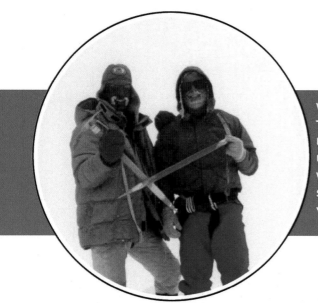

WERE THE DAY CLEAR I COULD SEE MT. MCKINLEY FROM
THE WINDOW...I PICTURE IN MY MIND ITS STUPENDOUS HEIGHT...
MANY HAVE ASSAILED ITS FLANKS; SOME HAVE PROCLAIMED
UNTRUTHS ABOUT IT; SOME HAVE CLIMBED BY GREAT EFFORT
WELL UP THE SLOPES; A VERY FEW, THE BEST BY NATURAL
SELECTION, HAVE REACHED THE SUMMIT AND ATTAINED THE BROAD
VISION DENIED THOSE AT LOWER ALTITUDES.

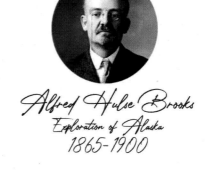

Alfred Hulse Brooks
Exploration of Alaska
1865-1900

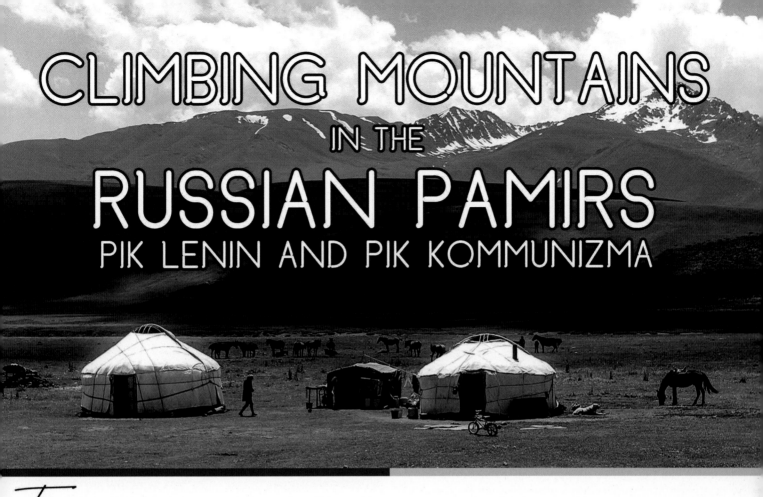

CLIMBING MOUNTAINS
IN THE
RUSSIAN PAMIRS
PIK LENIN AND PIK KOMMUNIZMA

*T*here are a lot of ways a guy can kill himself above 14,000 feet. I learned that in my climb of Denali in Alaska in 1986.

The four Japanese climbers that I saw dead and frozen solid on their ropes in the Japanese Couloir is still a haunting memory. Peering into a bottomless sparkling blue ice crevasse on the Kahiltna Glacier still gives me shivers. The avalanches, the accelerating falls on 30 degree slopes, the treacherous weather on any Denali climb can always bring on a shudder. All these memories give one a self-assured smugness that he was lucky to climb that mountain unharmed.

Nevertheless the lure of mountain climbing tends to gnaw at you so that by 1988 - specifically in July of 1988 - I had put aside the negatives of Denali and found myself on a Russian Aeroflot jet flying from Moscow to Soviet Central Asia to begin a mountain climbing expedition that was to include Pik Lenin at 23,500 feet and Pik Kommunizma at 24,500 feet.

During the long plane flight starting from Bakersfield to the Soviet Central Asian Republic of Kyrgesia I had plenty of time to think about why people climb mountains and specifically my own decision to climb again. I was now age fifty-one and had some second thoughts about what I was getting myself into.

Climbing offers a series of mental and physical challenges that are carried out in some of the most beautiful places on the planet. Overcoming those challenges, feeling the sense of accomplishment and learning more about yourself is tremendously rewarding.

For me the answer was very similar to why I had done the Ironman in Hawaii four times. Each time was more difficult, but each time you learned a little more about yourself and the experience was tremendously rewarding.

How does a trip such as this one to such a remote place as Soviet Central Asia begin? The seed is usually planted much earlier. For this trip the seed was Gary Bocade, the guide for my Denali climb in 1986. During our climb he kept practicing his Russian expressions - "Good morning. Good afternoon. How are you?" I climbed Denali with Gary in June 1986, but after the trip was concluded Gary traveled to Russia to climb in the Pamirs.

Gary was practicing his Russian expressions on our group. He had led a group of Russians on a successful climb of Denali, and they rewarded him by inviting him to climb at the Russian mountaineering encampment at Ashik-Tash in the Pamirs. Gary described the climb in the Pamirs as something totally different and unique even more than the Himalayas where he had also climbed.

Curiosity led me to seek some background about Pik Lenin and Pik Kommunizma. At that time in 1988 only a few Americans had ever been to the Pamirs. The Cold War was in full operation, and the Russians only allowed a few Americans to travel to Soviet Central Asia. The area had been closed to westerners essentially since the Russian Revolution in 1917. You had to be invited by the Russian Mountaineering Organization to climb in the Pamirs.

The Pamir Mountains are a mountain range in central Asia at the junction of the Himalayas where the Tian Shan, Karakoram and Hyndkush monstrous ranges converge, and the Pamirs have some of the world's highest mountains. The Pamirs run through the Asian Republics of Kyrgesia, Tagikistan and border Afghanistan. The word "pamir" is a geological term that refers to a flat plateau or u-shaped valley surrounded by mountains forming when a glacier or ice field melts leaving a rocky plain. There are many glaciers in the Pamir mountains. Two of the highest mountains in the Pamirs are Ismoil Somoni Pik which from 1962 to 1998 when I was there was called Pik Kommunizma glorifying communism, the political system of the Russian Republic. It is 24,590 feet. And Pik Lenin, named after the Russian Communist Revolutionary, had its name changed to Ibn Shina Pik. It is 23,300 feet. The Pamir mountains are covered in snow throughout most of the year and have a long and bitter cold winter and a short cool summer.

After we completed our Denali traverse in Alaska climbing up from the south side of the mountain to the top of Denali at 20,300 feet and then down the north side on the Muldrow Glacier to Wonder Lake in Denali National Park, a total of some 140 miles, Gary asked me if I would be interested in joining a climb he was putting together for the Russian Pamirs. Well, of course I would.

I had a heart-to-heart conversation with Gary and said, "Gary, I am now fifty-one years old. Should I be trying to climb a 25,000 foot-peak based upon your experience with me on Denali, could I do it?" Gary responded that he thought that I was in great condition, well-trained and should be able to handle all of the challenges.

Gary described the Pamirs as fantastically beautiful and challenging mountains - completely unexplored country for Americans. The area was mysterious, the home of the yeti, the endangered snow leopard, the rare astor markhor mountain goat and the kirqhiz, a nomadic horse people who lived on the Central Asian Steppes.

After Gary described the Pamirs I felt it was the kind of adventure I could not turn down, and I committed myself in January 1988 to being a member of the group. From January to June I spent the time again getting in peak physical condition and buying the necessary equipment that I would need for the trip.

For conditioning I followed my Ironman routine of biking 1,000 miles a month, running 40 miles a week and swimming 20,000 yards plus in a week in the pool in addition to gym workouts with my trainer.

As to equipment I had most of what I needed from the Denali climb, but a new Chouinard ice ax, super gaiters, a new jumar ascender, slings, figure eight, chest harness, and new crampons were added to the climbing assortment. I read as much as I could about the area.

The constant refining and redesigning in development of mountain climbing equipment is amazing. Such inventiveness goes into it. The last week before the trip which was to begin on Sunday, July 3, 1988 I spent packing and re-packing, winnowing down surplus equipment and only keeping what I absolutely needed; I would be carrying it all on my back at altitude.

I knew that I would have to carry everything, but it still seemed as if I had two to three of everything and that my bags must have weighed over 100 pounds. How will I ever carry this load plus my share of food, fuel and climbing gear up to 24,500 feet or higher? Oh well, I know most of it will be shed along the way.

Sunday, July 3, 1988: Catch a bus in Bakersfield to Los Angeles International Airport where I check in at the SAS Airlines for a 5:20 p.m. departure for Copenhagen.

My SAS plane flew from Los Angeles to Copenhagen, stopping briefly in Stockholm and then on to Helsinki, Finland from where I would fly to Moscow on July 5, 1988.

I arrived in Copenhagen, Denmark at 4:00 a.m., 1:00 p.m. Bakersfield time, and spent about an hour in the duty-free shop walking through the high quality and quantity goods.

I left Copenhagen at 2:00 p.m. local time arriving in Stockholm, Sweden fifty-five minutes later at 6:00 a.m., 4:00 p.m. Bakersfield time. I had time to relax in the airport café for a good meal.

At 7:45 p.m. I departed on SAS for Helsinki, Finland. The flight was smooth and uneventful arriving in Helsinki around 9:00 p.m. local time. I changed a few dollars to Finnish marks and passed through customs without any problems. I took the Finland bus into town arriving at the town terminal. My hotel was located next door.

Most people in Finland speak English; it's very easy to get around. I had dinner that night in the hotel café and hit the sack around 12:00 p.m. local time.

Monday, July 5, 1988: Up at 6:00 a.m. and off for a one hour run on a beautiful path around central Helsinki Lake where the 1952 Olympics were held in the stadium downtown. Paavo Nurmi, the great Finnish runner, ran the marathon that year. The running path was composed of wood chips which made easy footing, and it went through the woods, a beautiful run. I kept a 7 minute 30 seconds pace for about 10 miles, a wonderful workout in the cool Helsinki morning air.

After returning to the hotel I showered then walked around the city for about three hours up by the harbor, through the parks and the shopping district. Helsinki is a beautiful city, and there is a great deal to do.

At 12:00 noon I left on the bus for the Flag Station (airport) and at 2:10 p.m. boarded the Finnair flight for Moscow. The flight was smooth, and we landed at Sheremetyevo, the major Moscow terminal. I passed through customs easily. The Russians didn't even inspect my bags. There was a rather long wait for transportation; I had to wait for members of the Russian sports committee to meet me and clear me through the airport.

We took a bus from the airport and arrived in downtown Moscow at the Sports Hotel at 10:00 p.m. I was told that I was not expected until July 6, 1988 so I had to pay an additional 50 rubles extra for a late dinner.

After dinner I checked into my room which was pretty shabby with a single bed. During my stay it was questionable as to whether or not the shower and water faucets would work. The TV never worked, and the room lights were hit or miss. The craftsmanship that went into the tile laying, painting, plastering were like so may things in Russia - pretty shoddy. Oh well. It really did not matter since I only needed the bed to sleep in and wasn't there for a luxurious vacation.

Wednesday, July 6, 1988: All the alpinists gathered in the main dining room for breakfast. There I met Larry Hensen, a tax lawyer from New York City, who had been to the Pamirs on a mountain trip the year before.

His entire group came down with dysentery, and only one climber made it to the top of Pik Lenin. Larry was back for his second try with some of the same people who had organized the climb themselves. Larry had now lost all of his luggage and would join us when he was able to find his luggage or purchase replacement equipment.

I also met Royal Robbins, a well known U.S. mountain climber and mountain man as well as clothing manufacturer, on his way to Siberia for a river-rafting trip. The Russians were thinking of opening up their Siberian rivers for river-rafting tours and had invited Royal Robbins to check them out.

The Sports Hotel was the destination in Moscow for a great variety of athletes engaged in sporting events in Russia: basketball, soccer, tennis, weight lifting, mountain climbing, bicycling, running track and field, swimming. It was enjoyable interacting with all the different athletes and hearing their stories, their origins, what sport they were competing in.

For breakfast I was served sliced salami, cheese, heavy black coffee, rolls and jam. It did fill one up.

One of our Russian interpreters, Dana, took Larry Hensen and me on a tour of the Metro Subway to the central city. The subway or Metro in Moscow was quite impressive. Each station is magnificently decorated. We exited at Lenin's Library and had a good walk around the City Center to St. Catherine's Cathedral, Lenin's Tomb and downtown Moscow.

Larry, Dana and I spent most of the day in downtown Moscow, and by the time we got back to the hotel we were to meet the other climbers in our group at dinner. Our group was quite eclectic: Richard Goodell, a doctor from Phoenix, Arizona; Allan Ropp, a sound engineer from Cincinnati, Ohio; Fred Ziel, an endocrinologist from UCLA Medical School; David Bergenzer, a Utah school teacher; Stacey Tanniguchi, an Alaska teacher and our mountain guide. Our group seemed to be quite compatible from the beginning. All were obviously in good physical and mental condition for the trip and looking forward to climbing mountains in the Pamirs.

Thursday, July 7, 1988: We took a tour of the city with other climbers that were gathering for the trip to the Russian climbing camp at Ashik-Tash at 12,000 feet. Our touring group included climbers from Japan, Hungary, Bulgaria, France and Russia. We went to Red Square and witnessed the changing of the guard at Lenin's Tomb and toured the GUM Department store.

Dana, our guide, was quite political, and we had some lively discussions about U.S. versus U.S.S.R. relations.

I had been to Moscow in 1980 with a group of lawyers for a legal conference. Our guides on that trip were very zip-mouthed and did not have much to say. Dana, on the other hand, spoke animatedly without criticism of the great virtues of the U.S.S.R. She was, however, somewhat open-minded and wanted to know what people in the U.S.A. thought of the U.S.S.R. She expressed that perestroika could not work because the Russian economy and political system were too intertwined and people were afraid of change. She also expressed the opinion that Russian people did not really want to work that hard which was an interesting commentary on the psychological climate of the populace.

In contrast to the trip to Moscow ten years before there was now much more traffic, and people appeared better dressed and more prosperous. The buildings however were shabby, and nothing really worked except the Russian Army and the space program; except for those two programs Russia was still a third-world poor country.

We left the hotel at 10:00 p.m. and packed up with the group that we had toured with in Moscow - the Japanese, Bulgarians, Hungarians, Austrians. We were all transported to a different airport where we were told it would be a long wait and that we would not be taking off until around 2:30 a.m.

Just before we left we were driven to a lounge that opens onto the tarmac of the airport. Some of the members of our climbing groups were allowed to walk out on the tarmac and walk around the planes; most were Aeroflot jets. We were allowed to inspect them, even take pictures sitting on the wheels. It just seemed quite incredible in a country that at that time was so fanatical about security.

We departed Moscow at 2:30 a.m. and flew some 3,000 miles across Russia, landing in the Soviet Central Asia city of Osh, the capital of the Soviet Republic of Kirghiza, after a five hour flight through several time zones. The flight was a somber contrast to western aviation standards. The plane was packed full with no assigned seating; we boarded and took whatever empty seat we could find.

The plane was a large Aeroflot jet looking similar to a DC 10 with the engine in the tail section. The interior, however, was very crowded - three seats abreast on the each side of the aisle. Most of us were climbers with a tremendous amount of climbing gear and paraphernalia, and the plane was heavily loaded. Aside from the climbers the remainder of the seats were filled with Soviets on their way to Osh Kirghiza with a definite preponderance of Asian faces in the crowd. We flew east through five time zones, and when we arrived in

Osh we had a fourteen hours difference in time from Bakersfield. On 07/09/88 at 10:00 p.m. it was 11:00 p.m. on 07/08/88 in Bakersfield. In departing the plane at Osh, a major central Asian capital, we exited into a different time zone, a different world, a time from the past where we were greeted by young Kirghiz girls in native dress and men in their traditional Kirghiz headwear. Yes, we are in central Asia. Osh is an ancient city on the silk route from China.

As guests of the Russian Mountain Federation we were treated to an elaborate feast in the café upstairs at the airport - lavosh bread; mares milk - a heavy cream-like dairy product; curdled cheese; fresh local grapes; peaches; apples; pastries stuffed with cooked meat; peppers stuffed with meat; and then shish kebab - all served with dark aromatic thick coffee and crushed cherry juice. It was delicious and filling.

The geography around Osh is very similar to that of the southern San Joaquin Valley, my home - hot, arid, all irrigated, cotton, grapes, apples, peaches, corn. The living standards, however, are similar to those of rural Mexico. Much of the transportation was by tractors and other mechanical implements along with horse-drawn carts and wagons and bicycles. There were few private automobiles.

After the hearty lunch and a few patriotic speeches we left Osh in four-wheel drive buses. We started up the mountain valleys mostly on dirt or gravel roads, through alluvial stream beds that are running strong this time of the year.

The people are predominantly Asiatic: women in bright colorful native dress; men with goatskin hats. As we get higher up into the mountains we run into the nomadic tribes of Kirghiz who live in goatskin house tents or yurts and herd sheep on their horses. They used the roads, part gravel part asphalt, to herd their stock of goats and horses, and our buses had to maneuver around them. We get close glimpses of the natives from the bus windows - strong, sunbaked Asiatic people on horseback wearing goatskin or fur hats doing what their tribes have done for centuries - nomadic living in the high mountains of Central Asia. The bus ride is quite jolting and tiring on hard uncomfortable seats.

We climbed up to one pass at 12,000 feet where there was a large sculpture of a snow leopard guarding the pass. On another pass there was a sculpture of the rare central Asian astor markhor mountain goat.

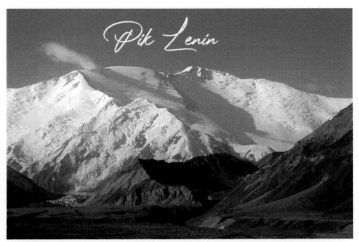

Pik Lenin

After many hours on the road we crossed from Kyrgystan into the Republic of Tajikistan where the villages become more primitive. The scenery becomes more spectacular with the dramatic Pamir range covered in white snow always in view. Some of the roads are scary, steep and winding and twisting down into deep river valleys. We cross streams with the water up to the tops of the four-wheel drive bus tires.

We have to pass through a guarded military checkpoint where the heavily-armed Russian soldiers stare at us steely-eyed and wonder why we are all there. After much discussion with our drivers and guides we were allowed to pass. The war just across the border in Afghanistan is waging against the Russians, and security is intense.

When we enter Tajikistan the Pamir range emerges spectacularly into view, lifting suddenly out of the green fertile valley without foothills almost like the Alaska range in Alaska. We can see Pik Lenin at 23,500 feet, an impressive sight. On the other side of the Pamirs is China.

The bus ride to Ashik-Tash was an exhausting twelve hours, the latter parts over rugged and dusty, steep trails where we could not travel more than five to ten miles per hour. We arrived at Ashik-Tash at 9:00 p.m. covered with dust and exhausted.

Ashik-Tash at 12,000 feet elevation is a large Russian mountaineering encampment in the Pamir range with portable dining rooms and kitchens, showers and latrines. It is assembled during the climbing season then dismantled in the winter when the area is covered with snow. There was a large goatskin yurt for drinking and conversation.

We were given space in the open, grassy meadow surrounding the camp to set up our tents. After hot showers we readily devoured a dinner of hot mashed potatoes, meat, hot tea and dessert. After dinner we hit the sack and slept soundly. Everyone was tired out from the long, hard bus ride.

Saturday, July 9, 1988: Up at 7:30 a.m. washing in the sparkling clear cold stream running down through the meadow by the camp. We were told not to drink the water without purification. We had breakfast in the dining hall with hot porridge, lavosh, hot Russian thick black aromatic coffee and rolls. The good life.

The day is spectacular. I am sitting in front of my tent without a shirt on at 12,000 feet in the warm bright sun looking up at Pik Lenin packed in glaciers and covered in snow. What a sight! It is both an awesome sight and intimidating. Pik Lenin, at 23,500 feet, is higher than I had ever been before. Can I do it? As I look around there are approximately one hundred or more tents that house mountaineers from all over the world, and as I sit and write in my journal alpinist people walk past speaking a variety of languages.

We are to attend a meeting with our Russian advisers today to finalize our plans for climbing - whether to climb Pik Lenin or Pik Kommunizma first. Our group meets at the camp headquarters building with Victor Baibara, a world-renowned Russian climber, for a very pleasant and helpful chat. Victor is the director of all of the Soviet sports camps in the Pamirs and gave us a warm welcome telling us that by opening their arms to us they could improve Soviet-American relations. Sasha Ivanoff, a very bright young man, helpful and pleasant with a good command of English is appointed as our interpreter. The Soviets seemed to be generally interested in our safety and welfare and told us they wanted to do all they could to make our trip a successful summit of both Lenin and Kommunizma.

With Victor we went over the details of our climb, what our approach to the mountains would be, how many days and what we could expect. Our plan was to climb Pik Lenin first. The Russian theory of climbing is "climb high, sleep low" to properly acclimate. We used the same theory in climbing Denali. Since Gary had climbed with the Russians he liked that idea. We double-carried everything up the Kahiltna Glacier. One day we would load up with our backpacks and sleds and climb all day, bury all of our equipment in the snow so that ravens wouldn't destroy it then go back down where we started, spend the night and the next day return with another half load to the same location. We spent fourteen days on the Kahiltna Glacier double-carrying all of our equipment. It was pure drudgery, but it paid off in acclimatization and strengthening at altitude.

Pik Lenin is 23,500 feet and is on the border of Tajikistan and Kyrgystan. It is the second highest mountain in the Pamir Mountains exceeded only by Pik Kommunizma.

Pik Lenin was discovered in 1871 and originally named Mt. Kaufmann after Constantine Kaufmann, the first governor general of Turkestan. In 1928 the mountain was renamed Lenin Pik after the Russian revolutionary Vladimir Lenin. There have been many attempts to change the name of the mountain after Soviet Central Asia withdrew from the Russia Federation in 2006. The newest name is Ibn Shina Pik.

After our meeting I took a hike in the afternoon to the Russian monument a few miles from camp where eight Soviet women were killed in a blizzard on Pik Lenin in 1974. This was a very lovely spot overlooking the valley where camp Ashik-Tash is located. There is also a monument nearby to all of the climbers who have been killed in the Pamirs. One monument was financed by the parents of an American climber that was killed there in a fall in the early 1980s.

After the hike and returning to camp I re-packed all my gear in my backpack. Our backpacks were to be flown by helicopter into Camp I so we could free climb from Ashik-Tash up to Camp I up the Lenin Glacier without heavy loads. Camp I is where the real climbing will begin.

Sunday, July 10, 1988: I was up early and packed and stored the equipment that I had brought on the trip that I would not be using on the Lenin climb.

We enjoyed a big Russian breakfast with porridge, bread, cheese, sausage, meat and potatoes combined like a hash and hot cocoa, delicious and filling.

Before leaving on the helicopter a Russian doctor examined our climbing crew and took our blood pressure. The doctor had me do ten quick knee bends and then took my blood pressure again. The doctor said he was amazed that I was in superb condition. I was fifty-one.

We got underway with just light backpacks at 10:00 a.m., leaving on a dirt mountain trail out of Ashik-Tash. The initial hike up through the valley was beautiful with lush green meadows abundant with white, yellow, purple wildflowers. It was a delightful hike - with just a day pack. The first part of our climb was up a glacial moraine on dirt trails where we eventually crossed over onto the Lenin Glacier. Some of the initial glacier hiking was easy-going in hiking boots, but as we started getting up higher the snow was showing the effects of the high mountain sun-some of it "rotting" and soft. We kept falling into knee-deep holes filled with ice water. Our hiking boots were wet, our feet cold and miserable.

We had only a few quick stops from 10:00 a.m. and continued the rest of the day until we arrived at Camp I around 4:30 p.m., very tired since we moved at a very fast pace. I had a headache from the elevation gain. The Russians told us that the elevation at Camp I is about 14,200 feet, but overall the altitude effects were not too bad. On Mt. Denali elevation effects at 14,000 feet were quite noticeable, but here we are closer to the equator and there is better oxygen.

The sun was merciless on the trip to Camp I, and even though I wore protective hat gear, glacier goggles and I coated with sunscreen, my face was red and puffy and my eyes hurt. After some hot cocoa, soup and dinner I felt much better, my headache waning. We would have more glacier climbing tomorrow and I would really have to protect my head, face and eyes. I had high elevation goggles and face protection masks that I could wear to protect from the piercing sun.

Our climbing plan was to carry our equipment and backpack loads to Camp II at 16,800 feet and then return to sleep at Camp I. As I indicated the Russian theory of climbing was to climb high and sleep low in order to properly acclimate. Gary Bocade, our Denali guide as I said, used the Russian method on Denali which I think was a major reason why we were in the small percentage of climbers who actually make it to the summit of Denali. By the time we were over 14,000 feet on Denali we had slept at low elevations seven or eight times and were well acclimated.

After relaxing I noticed my back was stiff and painful, and I was not looking forward to the next day which promised to be rougher.

Before we had dinner, Victor Baivara came over to talk to us. He had followed us up the glacier often making suggestions as to a route. There were some tricky places on the glacier, open crevasses and streams that had cut water stream channels in the glacier that were quite deep, tricky and dangerous to get across. Victor only speaks a few words of English but knows the mountain extremely well and was able to point out the best routes for us to follow up the glacier. He climbs it frequently in the summer.

Victor is a master climber and holds the prestigious position in the Russian alpine world of snow leopard. A person can achieve a snow leopard status by climbing the highest mountains in the Soviet Union. A snow leopard is equivalent to being a professional athlete in the U.S.A. Victor was also involved in the rescue of the bodies of the Soviet women who were killed on Pik Lenin in 1974. He was a good friend of a Soviet climber whose wife was one of the women who was killed in the tragedy. Victor genuinely likes Americans and likes to be around them; he told us enthusiastically about his climb of Denali in Alaska with Gary Bocade. After the meeting with Victor it was 8:30 p.m. and I was tired and left to get in my sleeping bag.

Monday, July 11, 1988: I woke early, we packed up the camp and were out on the trail by 8:30 a.m It was still very cold. Our plan was to carry a heavy load to Camp II at 16,800 feet, cache the load and return to sleep at Camp I. The climb up the glacier was slow, steep and steady. The sun was again frying-pan hot, reflecting off of the snow. I covered myself with sunblock and wore a kerchief on my head with a hat. I had forgotten what drudgery climbing up a glacier can be when you have to double-carry everything. Here though we were not roped but clearly followed in line the climber in front. We arrived at Camp II, cached our supplies by burying them in the snow and retraced our steps back down to Camp I. Downhill was much faster, and we arrived at Camp I at 5:00 p.m. after only two and a half hours. This day I can definitely feel the effects of altitude with headache and fatigue, thoroughly tired and can't wait to eat and go to sleep. Our plan, however, is to try to get up as early as possible and try to leave camp all packed at 6:00 a.m. to avoid the boiling sun.

Tuesday, July 12, 1988: It rained quite heavily last night but we were well protected in our tents. It rained for several hours; this is wild weather country: cold in the morning, searing hot during the day and rain or snow at night. We were all up at 4:00 a.m. The rain had stopped and it was still dark and we packed up our gear using our headlamps and left camp at 6:00 a.m., just as it was starting to get light. Back up on the glacier and through the worst part by 9:00 a.m. The surface was frozen and icy so we used crampons. We made good time and got to Camp II at 11:30 a.m. The last few miles I had a headache and was dizzy and fatigued. Carrying supplies up a glacier is a grunt. At Camp II we unpacked and set up camp, and by this time the sun was out and hot. We sought relief from the sun in our tents.

Wednesday, July 13, 1988: According to Victor's plan we took a rest day at Camp II at 16,800 feet. I did not sleep well last night - had trouble breathing and would awake in a start trying to catch my breath. Also during the night I was plagued with bad dreams. All this is no doubt due to the decrease in oxygen affecting the brain. We have a change in plans. Victor - who was still guiding our climbing - recommended that we go to Camp III at 20,000 feet, sleep the night and then return all the way down to Camp I for proper acclimatization. We all argued with Victor about his plan since we would go almost to the summit and then go all the way back down to sleep again before going to the top. He thought this would be good training for our climb on Pik Kommunizma which we were to

climb following Lenin. We finally compromised and decided that we would carry equipment to Camp III, sleep there and return only to Camp II the following day and night and then return again to Camp III before starting the push for the summit. The sun is blazing hot again today, and my thought was that it had to be having effects on the glaciers. The location of Camp II is really exposed to avalanche paths and is a concern to me and to my fellow climbers. I had enough experience in the Alaska mountains and in the Sierra Nevadas to know avalanche danger. I will be glad to get out of here and leave this camp tomorrow. Because of the change of plans we spent the day building two igloos-cutting out large blocks of frozen snow and making a shelter to protect us from the sun. We did not build an ice roof over the igloos but used a tarp. Sleeping in the igloo was warm and comfortable. However, it did snow most of the night.

Thursday, July 14, 1988: It snowed all night, at times heavily, and we had a good accumulation of snow on the ground and up on the glacier. The plan was to leave camp at 7:00 a.m., but that did not materialize because of the storm and poor visibility. The plan now was to wait out the storm and see what happens.

That night I took a Diamox tablet 250 mgs which is supposed to help breathing in high altitude. I was experiencing apnea and shortness of breath. That night I did not sleep very well and felt claustrophobic in the igloo. Everyone in our climbing group appeared to be healthy accept for apnea and headache. No other severe altitude reactions. It was snowing off and on all morning with poor visibility so we continued to wait. Around noon the weather broke, the snow stopped and we decided to take a load up the trail hopefully to Camp III and cache it and return to sleep at Camp II. Immediately out of Camp II is a very steep climb up a 30 or 40 degree icy glacier. It had stairsteps in it from previous climbers. The climb with crampons was a slow steady pace. I was feeling pretty good. The slope, however, did not change and continued relentlessly up a ridge, and as we got on the edge of the ridge the wind started up and really blasted us. On the exposed ridge the temperature dropped considerably and visibility became very poor. Instead of going all the way to 20,000 feet at Camp III we decided to cache the supplies at 18,000 feet and return tomorrow. The return trip back down to Camp II was fast.

After we returned to Camp II the snow continued to fall, at times quite heavily. For dinner that night we had a Mountain Trip beef (i.e., rehydrated) stroganoff which was much appreciated by all. The plan tomorrow is to head for Camp III weather permitting. At 7:00 p.m. I am tired and get in my sleeping bag. It is still snowing.

Friday, July 15, 1988: Up at 6:00 a.m. It is still snowing and socked in - not much visibility. We decide we have to go up anyway and then just follow the stairsteps that we had created in the last two days. We get away from camp by 9:15 a.m. with light snow, about two miles of visibility. I feel rested today because last night I got some good sleep. The climb back to Camp III is long, steep and difficult. In addition, there is two feet of snow that covered the trail we left before. We must just plow through the new snow and the going is tough. The course again is steep, never letting up. We actually get to 20,000 feet but descend back down to 19,600 feet where we have more protection from the weather and set up camp. Everyone is really tired. Even though we are at almost 20,000 feet there is not much of a view. It is very cloudy and snowing. If it does clear up there should be spectacular views of the Pamirs from here. In the tent I am very tired. I will eat and then go to bed. The route up to Camp IV rises right out of Camp III, and it looks steep and formidable. However, if we reach Camp IV tomorrow we only have a four hour climb to the summit.

Saturday, July 16, 1988: Last night the wind blew fiercely most of the night at times causing the stays on the tent to squat down, the top of the tent coming down onto our faces. I thought several times that the tent was going to be blown away and made contingency plans to grab certain clothes to put on in case the tent was blown away. This was the worst weather that we had had. The wind did not let up and blew steadily until about 8:00 a.m. when it suddenly stopped. By 9:00 a.m. the wind was down to periodic bursts. The sun actually came out and it was rather pleasant. The views now were spectacular. Our plan now was to carry everything to Camp IV, cache it and then return to sleep at Camp III again tonight.

We left Camp III around 11:00 a.m. for Camp IV, climbed up through a rocky ridge mostly frozen in ice with okay footing with crampons. The wind picked up considerably toward the top of the ridge and at this elevation was extremely cold. I had on my pile pants and long underwear and outer wind pants. I could still feel the icy wind piercing through my outer garments onto my legs. I had on a face mask and my warmest wool pile hat but was still freezing cold. I remembered being on Denali at 18,000 feet for two days in 60 degree below 0 and it gave me courage that I could do this.

We arrived at Camp IV at 2:45 p.m. and spent an hour or so building a platform for sleeping. We set up our tent behind an ice block wall for protection. The elevation at Camp IV is 20,400 feet, so this was a new altitude record for me. I did not feel as bad at this altitude as I did on Denali.

Denali is the northern-most 7,000 meter peak in the world and only 200 miles from the arctic circle so oxygen is less available at that latitude than at the same elevation near the equator. There is more oxygen available at the equator at the same altitude. The Pamirs are on the same latitude as Portland, Oregon and Denali is only 200 miles from the arctic circle. Breathing was easier in the Pamirs.

On the return trip back to Camp III Stacey Tanniguchi, our guide, fell through a snowy crust into a crevasse down to his shoulders. He was hanging with his ice ax. Since I was right in front of him I was able to pull him out with my ice ax without any injury or mishap. On the return to Camp III the wind had died down and we were covered with a slight mist but the sun was able to penetrate and it was pleasant climbing. All of our group were in good spirits and looking forward to tomorrow when the plan was to move everything to Camp IV and then make the summit attempt.

On Denali at this altitude everyone was obviously suffering from the effects of altitude: nausea, headache, shortness of breath and general intolerance toward others. If the weather holds up we can summit Pik Lenin in 2 days.

Sunday, July 17, 1988: I have been gone now two weeks and sure miss my wife, my family and my two little cocker spaniel doggies Blondie and Blossom.

Unfortunately last night the wind again blew violently all night and the tent felt again as if it were coming apart. The ridge for Camp III is exposed to the full blast of the wind from the west. It was also extremely cold and I did not sleep much that night.

At 3:00 a.m. I had to take a potty break and got out of the tent. The sky was crystal clear, and the skies were absolutely brilliant with no impurities in the air. The big dipper was in the western sky, and I felt as if I could reach up and grab it. In the eastern sky Venus looked like a large lightbulb suspended just above the horizon; it almost looked artificial. I had never seen Venus look so bright and so near. The next morning after a leisurely breakfast of hot oatmeal we were packed up and headed back to Camp IV. The climb up was more difficult this time since my pack was heavier and the wind was blowing relentlessly and piercingly cold. Even with all my cold weather gear I was still very cold. The cold wind zapped my energy and strength more than anything.

We arrived back at Camp IV at 2:30 p.m., the day bright and sunny but very windy and very cold. Camp was all set up and we were in two tents - three per tent - resting and sleeping for the summit push tomorrow.

We should be successful in making the summit unless the weather or sickness intervenes.

On the radio check at 9:00 p.m. we received disquieting news; a big storm was due tonight or tomorrow. This caused quite a bit of consternation among the group. Several were in favor of packing early and going down, others wanted to stay. We were advised not to try the summit with the approaching storm. Our Russian advisors knew the mountain better than any of us, and we respected their advice. At 20,000 feet we did not want to expose ourselves to unpredictable danger. At this elevation the weather is always an unpredictable wild card and you have to rely on those with more experience.

Monday, July 18, 1988: The wind blew on and off all night, at times gale force. Again the tents were in jeopardy. It was bitter cold with lots of blowing spindrifts invading everything. It was uncomfortable and cold in the tents. David said he wanted to go back since we had only one more dinner and we discovered that neither of the stoves worked. Stacey, our guide, said we would have to eat cold dry food for the climb to the summit. Everyone was agreeable to that, and I thought the consensus was we would go for the summit tomorrow. I was ready. However, Alan Ropp said he was not going to go for several reasons: 1) there was no food other than for one night; 2) we were advised not to try the summit in the approaching storm; 3) neither stove worked and we could not have hot drinks; 4) some of our group were too slow. Stacey Tanniguchi, our guide, said if one did not go then his decision would be that everyone would not go. We would never split the group. Since he was the guide we all agreed before the trip started that his decision would be the deciding factor. Rick was very upset because this would be his only chance to summit. He traveled all the way to Russia and Soviet Central Asia and we are now at the last camp and within a few hours of the summit. There were some hard words exchanged.

Stacey said that he would take into consideration everybody's view but based upon all the circumstances it was his decision that we would go down. We packed up and started down. There were still strong winds and clouds. We arrived at Camp III in one and a half hours and headed on back down to Camp II. As we approached Camp II the weather improved.

At Camp II we picked up our cache that we had previously left there and everyone was very heavily loaded. We headed on down to Camp I arriving there at 5:00 p.m. The nature of the glacier changed considerably since we started our trip. The crevasses had widened. There were more ice holes in the glacier surface and more stream cutting through the glacier which made it quite dangerous. At Camp I we were invited to dinner by the Russian coaches. At this camp we had an interpreter, Yuri, so that we could exchange conversation. Yuri is a strong personality and entertaining. He introduces us to Sashi, a young Soviet doctor, and we have dinner in their hut. Dinner is very pleasant with pleasant conversation covering the topics of climbing in the U.S.S.R.; climbing in Alaska; medicine in the U.S.A. and U.S.S.R.; earnings in both countries; customs, etc. All of us enjoyed the conversations. The Russians were very amicable, open and friendly. Since we had an interpreter we were all understood and the experience was good for all of us.

Tuesday, July 19, 1988: Slept at the Russian camp last night. Slept incredibly well. I could feel the rich oxygen flowing through my lungs even though I am still at 14,200 feet. It was an almost euphoric feeling.

I packed up with a light pack. All of my heavy gear I again left for the helicopter to bring back to the main camp. We started our trek back down over the glacier to base camp. Yuri led. He has long legs and set a furious pace and had us almost running down the glacier. When we came to the end of the glacier we climbed a very steep slippery path over the pass of travelers. Ordinarily I would be huffing and puffing but now charged up the steep incline with great leg strength and no loss of breath feeling in great physical condition.

We returned to base camp at 2:00 p.m. and had a great Russian lunch of thick vegetable soup, rice, meat, fresh tomatoes, thick dark Russian red hot tea and fresh grapes - heavenly food after the dehydrated food. We all overindulged.

The next big treat was a nice hot shower where I scrubbed with shampoo from the Park Lane Hotel in New York and conditioner from Aspen Square in Colorado that I had in my dopp kit. Some combination. I spent the remainder of the day washing clothes, relaxing, napping and waiting for the helicopter to return our equipment from Camp I.

Back at base camp there was some grumbling among our group that we didn't make the last push to the summit. We were so close and within hours of the summit. However, there was the issue of the storm and the Russian advisors' superior experience on the mountain. We had all agreed from the outset that the guide would make the call as to whether or not to go to the summit. We had that same experience on Denali. There we were stuck at 18,000 feet for two days in bitter cold, 60 below 0, and Gary Bocade thought we would have to go down without summiting. However, as luck would have it we got break in the weather and

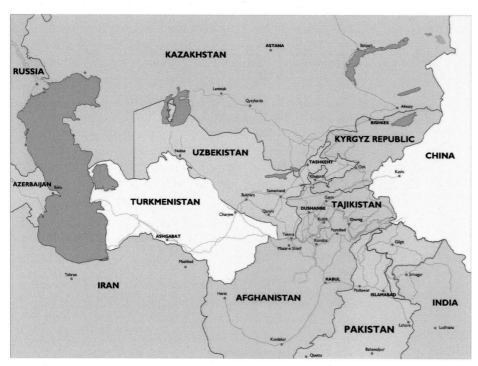

I must pause however to skip ahead to illustrate the great danger of climbing these high mountains.

On July 18, 1990 after I had returned from the climbing trip in the Pamirs I read in the *New York Times* of a horrible tragedy that had occurred on Pik Lenin at Camp II. One of the worst tragedies in the history of mountain climbing claimed the lives of at least forty members of international climbing teams that were killed on Friday, July 18, 1990 by an avalanche that buried Camp II. Camp II was called "The Frying Pan" because of the heat that could accumulate in the high mountain altitude.

were able to get to the summit in that situation. Looking back now on the experience and what later happened on Pik Kommunizma I can't second-guess Stacey. It is too easy to get one's ego involved and not take an overall view of the situation. In retrospect I have to agree that Stacey made the right decision although I am extremely disappointed we did not make the summit. I felt I was ready physically and mentally to go to the summit.

Wednesday, July 20, 1988: Back at base camp and life is leisurely and slow-paced again. There are three huge meals a day and we begin sorting out our equipment and planning for a climb of Pik Kommunizma. Stacey is ordering and arranging our food supplies. Our evenings are spent at the yurt. We renew our relationship with Mats and Duren who were both members of the Swedish Armed Special Forces. We met them on Lenin at Camp IV where we were camped on a ridge exposed to the weather. These two guys were two of the toughest men I have ever met. They did summit Lenin. They spent the night of July 19, 1988 sleeping in a snow cave by our camp, got up at night and with headlights made the summit. They had no protection from the weather other than the snow cave and slept in the cold weather gear that they had brought in their packs. These were extremely tough guys.

In the yurt we had great conversations with the Swedes and the other climbers of various nationalities especially with the use of Yuri, our interpreter. The two Swedes spoke excellent English and were able to help with all of the conversations as they did speak other languages.

We were scheduled to depart on Thursday, July 21, 1988 by helicopter to the base of Pik Kommunizma to begin our climb of that spectacular mountain.

The victims included twenty-seven Soviet climbers - I am sure some of the Soviet climbers that we met were involved. Leonard Troshchinenko, one of the Soviet's leading climbers, was killed in the avalanche. The dead included six Czech climbers, four Israelis, two Swiss and a Spaniard. No Americans were involved.

The report from the *New York Times* indicated that an earth tremor destabilized a massive avalanche of snow and debris which cascaded down the 30 degree slope and fell onto Camp II burying them under mountains of snow. The Frying Pan camp had been used for six decades by climbers pausing in their ascent of Lenin Pik. The news report indicated that deep snow was hindering rescue efforts and it would be months before all bodies could be recovered. Climbing and rescue specialists from the Pamir region rushed to the scene to search for victims, and other specialists were flown out from Moscow.

As I said earlier I always had an eerie feeling at Camp II - The Frying Pan - since it was so exposed to steep mountains on three sides. There are many ways to kill oneself above 14,000 feet.

Thursday, July 21, 1988: Up early and packing to leave Ashik-Tash. Breakfast was melted cheese on toast, sausage and canned pineapple juice. We leave camp at 10:00 a.m. on an Aeroflot helicopter. These helicopter rides were usually white knucklers. The Aeroflot helicopters were left over from the Soviet World War II Air Force and made me wonder when stepping into the crew cabin as to whether this would be my last ride. The helicopters were old, rattled and shook as we flew over mountains at 15,000 feet.

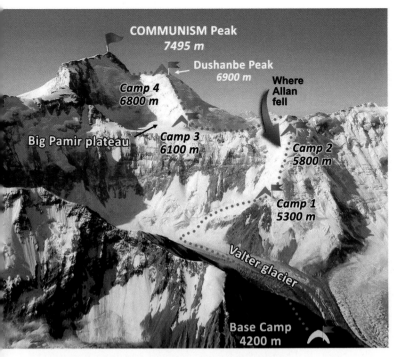

The helicopter flight from Ashik-Tash to the new camp at Moskvina at 13,800 feet can only be described by a string of superlatives - fantastic, incredible, awesome! All these words do not begin to do justice to the magnificent scenery that we passed over in the Pamir range flying from Pik Lenin to Pik Kommunizma from Ashik-Tash to Moskvina. Jagged peaks and ridges covered in snow and packed with glaciers. Snow and ice everywhere in an immense wilderness on the roof of the world.

We landed at Moskvina which is 13,800 feet and higher than Camp I on Lenin. The minute we land and exit the helicopter we see Pik Kommunizma which looms up from the camp - right there. So very intimidating especially the first half. Almost 11,000 feet of vertical elevation gain. As you look up the mountain you can see the route that you would have to take to get to the top.

It looks steep, high, scary and intimidating.

After landing we spent some time putting up our tents and organizing our gear. We had another huge Russian lunch - thick fish soup and vegetables served along with meatballs, potatoes and fresh tomatoes and onions with Russian bread and lemonade. This was followed by fresh watermelon with red seeds. The Russians fed us extremely well.

In the afternoon we met with the Soviet climbing coach Borodokin, also a snow leopard, the originator of Borodokin Route to the top of Pik Kommunizma. He not only climbed it many times but had the route named after him. Borodokin was a very pleasant fellow who had been to Alaska and wanted to know where we all were from in the United States. There was not a word of propaganda from Borodokin - if anything much self-deprecation Russian versus U.S. climbing abilities. The Russians had set up a seasonal camp at Moskovin with even a commissary with tables and benches. That evening we had another heavy Russian dinner.

Friday, July 22, 1988: Up early and packed with our backpacks full and out on the trail. We followed a dirt trail along a stream up through the glacier from which it originated. There we put on our crampons. It was a long climb up an ice ramp and then up through approximately 1,000 feet on rock outcrops. We arrived at Camp I at about 3:00 p.m. It was cloudy, windy and very cold. We secured all the equipment we could in a cache and started back down carefully because it was very steep, rocky and slippery. We returned to base camp around 6:00 p.m. after about nine hours of climbing up and back. I was tired. However, I did take a bath in a bathing tent by the creek. It was set up with a stove to heat water, I was able to get a warm bath which was much appreciated.

That evening we had another robust Russian dinner which we readily consumed because we were all very hungry from the nine hours of climbing. The Russian coaches were talking about opening up a new climbing camp in the north near Pik Peabody which is on the border with China in the Tengian Mountains. I finally got into my sleeping bag about 9:30 p.m. and slept very soundly.

Saturday, July 23, 1988: Woke up with fresh snow falling and covering the ground. After breakfast it was still snowing.

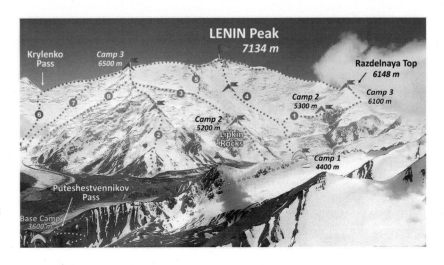

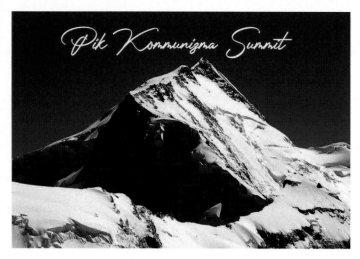

Pik Kommunizma Summit

Rick Goodell, one of our climbing partners, will be leaving us today and returning to Ashik-Tash and then Moscow. He expects to be back in Arizona by July 27, 1988. Rick is a doctor and had to return. We are now five climbers. Our plan was to return to Camp I. It was still snowing when we left and very cold. We left base camp at 9:45 a.m. in the snowstorm. As we climbed up the glacier the snow increased and then continued to fall the remainder of the day, at times heavily. As we climbed back up the glacier ramp we could hear the roar of avalanches from the steep cliffs on the face of Pik Kommunizma. We were not in the path of any of these avalanches coming off the cliffs. We then climbed back up through the rocky outcroppings which were now covered with snow. Some places were easier than the day before and some more difficult.

We arrive at Camp II at around 3:00 p.m., and set up camp in steadily falling snow. We were all sharing one tent. The Russians communicated to us that the weather reports indicated more snow both tonight and tomorrow and then four good days of weather. We will see. The elevation at Camp II is approximately 16,800 feet. We were told that our hardest day may be tomorrow in the climb from Camp II to Camp III. There were now five of us in our tent and we cooked dinner. The small burner did warm up the interior of the tent.

Sunday, July 24, 1988: It snowed all night, and we heard the constant roar of major avalanches coming off the steep cliffs of Pik Kommunizma. We were safe from any avalanche where we were camped on the ridge; however, the avalanches that did come off of the cliffs did run down onto the ramp that we were climbing yesterday. Because of the steepness the snow was very unstable. We woke up to clear skies and a bright sun, and we tried to lay out our equipment so that the sun would dry it out. Our plan was to continue up the ridge and try to make Camp III at 21,000 feet. The accumulation of snow and the avalanche danger caused all of us great concern. Our

camp was on a sharp ridge that had steep slopes on both sides falling away several thousand feet. As indicated we planned to carry our entire load from Camp II to Camp III. We were all in good condition and fully acclimated from climbing on Lenin for nine days. A group of five Russians who had camped right near us joined us and spent much of the morning visiting and talking with us and sharing hot tea. Some of them did speak some English, and they were very interesting people.

I had great admiration for the Russian climbers. Their equipment was ancient. They were climbing with leather boots and crampons that were held together with leather straps. Their tents did not even have zippers for closing but had loops with buttons. Their tents were heavy, ancient and made of waterproof canvas. Their clothing was also something you would see in a post-Korean War surplus store - old with holes and worn and patched. However, they were great climbers and made up for the lack of modern designer-labeled equipment with great strength, perseverance and agility. They were excellent athletes. We were slow on getting packed up and dressing, probably deliberately because we wanted the Russians to go in front of us and break trail. There was lots of fresh snow above us, and it would be difficult to be the first group out in those kinds of conditions, having to break a trail in loose snow. The Russians did leave in front of us. There were five of them. As the Russians went up I noted that all of them had their crampons on. It was not until approximately 10:00 a.m. that we were finally ready to start up the ridge. The path that we were going to take continued up for several thousand feet above us on a sharp ridge which rose very steeply with sheer drops in both directions. On Denali we would have been roped.

As we started to leave our tent platform Fred went first followed by David and then Stacey. Allan Ropp and I were standing on the platform and I said, "Go ahead, Allan. I am much slower." Allan said, "No. You go. I've got a heavy load. I will be slow today."

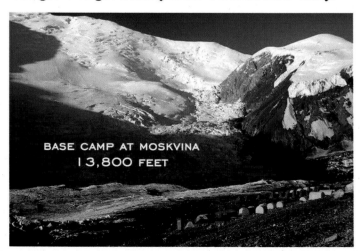

BASE CAMP AT MOSKVINA
13,800 FEET

We were all carrying heavy loads between fifty to sixty pounds as we planned to move the camp entirely up to Camp III without returning to Camp II. Allan Ropp was a small person, but he always carried his share or more of the load. I do not know exactly how much his pack weighed, but I could tell he was heavily loaded as we started up the ridge. The Russians had stamped out a good path for us to follow, and it was just a matter of putting one foot in front of the other in the same foot-holds that the Russians had stamped out. It was a good ploy to have let the Russians go first. For the first few hundred feet it was fairly routine going. Stacey, Allan and I were almost in lockstep with one another. That is my foot would go into the hole that Stacey's foot had just left, and Allan was doing the same immediately behind me. After a few hundred feet the ridge steep-ened considerably and we were climbing on a slope that was approximately 45 to 50 degrees. You could see that the ridge up in front of us continued in the same manner for several thousand feet.

After climbing approximately an hour and several hundred feet we came to what is called a fixed rope. The fixed rope was approximately 150 feet long and came to a point where it was secured into a second fixed rope. This rope had been put in by the Russians to assist climbers both going up and going down because the slope had steepened and was becoming very slippery. Up until this time the new snow was approxi-mately one foot deep but in places now the snow was not quite as deep because the wind had blown it off the surface underneath. The ice underneath was very slippery. At this point I noticed that Allan had fallen back off of my pace probably ten yards. I also looked around and noticed that Allan was slipping occasion-ally. In other words he was not getting a good foot purchase or grip. Allan was also using his ski poles at this time and had his ice ax strapped on his back. I was using crampons and an ice ax as were our other members. At about this point I looked back again and saw that Allan had attached onto the first fixed line with his jumar. A jumar is device used to hook onto a fixed rope to prevent a climber from falling. If he does fall the jumar, which is attached to the rope and then attached to his climbing belt and harness, will hold him in place or arrest a fall. I remember there was a Russian coming up behind Allan who was shouting to Allan, "Put on your crampons." This was the first indi-cation that I had that Allan was not wearing crampons. I didn't notice that he did not have them on at the time we left the camp because his feet were hidden in the fresh snow.

Crampons are a traction device usually with sharp pointed prongs that are attached to climbing boots to anchor a climber to an icy surface and prevent slipping. Crampons came in many different designs but the more modern versions are made of lightweight aluminum.

They are an essential gear for climbing on ice or hard packed snow.

I came to the point where the ropes were tied together and there was a large knot and some snow picks which are in the snow to secure the ropes. If a climber is using a jumar it is necessary at this point to un-hook the jumar, put it on the top side of the knot of the upper rope and continue up the rope. At this time I was still using my crampons and also my ice ax in my right hand. I was holding onto the rope with my gloved left hand to steady myself and give myself support.

At a point just above the transition between the two fixed ropes I heard a noise. I turned around and saw Allan spread eagle on the snow, stomach down, back pack in place, sliding very slowly down the slope toward a snow gully. My first thought was that Allan would be able to stop himself since he was sliding so slowly. It did look as if he was attempting to self-arrest or stop himself by digging his hands into the slope. Had he had his ice axe out he probably could have self-arrested because of his slow sliding.

I shouted to Stacey who was approximately two yards ahead of me, "Allan is falling."

Unfortunately Allan then began to pick up speed still on his stomach and then began to tumble sideways and bounce down the icy gully and then began to tumble uncontrollably like a rag doll . From where I was posi-tioned I could see him going the entire way down the icy gully until he came to a stop on a snow runout at the bottom of the gully. He had fallen approximately 1,500 feet with great speed.

By this time Dave and Fred had been alerted by Stacey. We all started back down the fixed line toward Camp II as fast as we could go. When we got to Camp II we jettisoned all of the food and fuel so that we would have a lightened load. We could not go directly down to Allan since it was too steep and dangerous. We had to return on the same route we had come up and then try to maneuver or traverse around to him. Allan never moved. Stacey and Fred left Camp II and started down the ridge as fast as they could go to try to get to Allan. There were also some other Russians down below who saw Allan fall and headed down on their way to him. Dave and I stayed at Camp II with our radio attempting to call base camp to get a doctor and helicopter up to the glacier some 1,000 feet below Allan. Allan fell at 11:47 a.m. - I looked at my watch when he fell.

It took approximately forty-five minutes before Stacey and Fred were able to reach Allan. The Russians had apparently gotten there first and did their best to give him whatever first-aid they could. The Russians, Stacey and Fred then put Allan in his sleeping bag in an attempt to insulate him against shock and made a makeshift stretcher out of one of the tents. They were able to haul Allan down approximately another 1,000 feet to the big glacier where the helicopter could land and reach him. Allan was alive but badly injured and unconscious. In the meantime the base camp had been alerted, and a woman doctor from the camp started up to meet the group that was coming down. The base camp doctor arrived approximately two hours after Allan's fall with medical supplies. She immediately hooked him up to an IV unit and gave him a series of injections the nature of which I do not know. A barricade was rigged up to protect Allan from the sun and he was left in his sleeping bag. He was unconscious, blood was coming from his nose and ears, and it was very obvious that he had been seriously injured. He did not respond to sound or any stimulus.

After David and I came down we found Allan's pack at the bottom of the snow ramp and brought it back to where he was located. Allan had his ice ax attached to the back of the pack. The ice ax has a carbon fiber shaft, and it was bent almost completely in two. There was also a stainless steel 2 ½ to 3 gallon cooking pot strapped to the back of the pack that had been smashed completely. This gave us some idea of the tremendous force involved in Allan's fall and that he had collided with rocks as he tumbled downward. Fred Zeal, who is a doctor, and the Russian doctor were also amazed that Allan had survived the fall because of the tremendous forces that were involved. Fred doubted Allan would live. At approximately 6:00 p.m. that afternoon a helicopter was able to reach Allan and fly him to Osh. Fred and Stacey wanted to accompany Allan, but the Russians would not let them go. After Allan was taken to Osh we had very little information as to what was going on. We went back to the Moskvina Camp and the next day were flown back to Ashik-Tash. We wired the American Embassy and told them what had happened and requested that they contact Allan's parents. We received very little information after that as to what was happening; we did not become aware until much later that the parents had in fact been notified by the American Embassy.

Wednesday, July 27, 1988: We got word from the Russian doctors that they gave Allan a 50/50 chance of survival. They were encouraged that his vital signs were good. However, Fred Zeil was more pessimistic and felt that unless Allan could be transferred to a major medical center his survival was doubtful. We still had not heard anything from the American Embassy as to what plans they had for helping Allan and his parents. Allan had fallen on Sunday, July 24, 1988. On a pre-arranged program we were not scheduled to leave Ashik-Tash for another nine days or until

August 2, 1988. Because of the inflexibility of the Russians we were not allowed to amend our program and leave earlier.

We tried to make the remaining stay as good as we could with the tragedy of Allan's fall always on everyone's mind. Allan's fall was unfortunate, but there were many things that could have prevented it:

1. Wearing crampons;
2. Being attached to the fixed rope with a jumar;
3. Having an ice ax out for self-arrest;
4. Being all roped together.

None of these safety precautions were in place at the time of Allan's fall. Yes, there are a lot of ways to kill oneself above 14,000 feet, but the risk is reduced when you have safety measures in place. When we returned to base camp we learned about another accident on Pik Lenin where two German climbers were found wondering aimlessly on Pik Lenin by the Russian coaches. One German had badly frostbitten hands and the other was suffering from altitude sickness. We saw the Germans in the yurt and the sight of the one with his frostbitten hands was shocking.

On July 27th I took a long hike from 10:00 a.m. to 2:30 p.m. up the canyon to a peak called the 19th Congress, a very rugged and beautiful area where three glacial rivers merge turning the outgoing stream into a tomato red color probably from the iron in the rock and soil. One river was a gray color, the third clear and clean and the middle river tomato red which caused the merged river to become red and to run with considerable volume.

On Thursday, July 28, 1988 David and I hiked up the canyon to the east of the camp leaving around 10:00 a.m., hiking over a pass around 12:00 noon. There we ate some cookies and returned to camp by 2:00 p.m. We had a great climb and were feeling in good condition. The same day Sasha, our guide, took David, Fred, Stacey and me on a hike to a Kyrgyzstan encampment where we encountered a Kyrgyzstan family at their yurt. We were invited into the yurt by the patron. Inside the yurt it was very clean and elaborately decorated with Asian carpets and wall hangings. The yurt was heated by a small stove in the center of the yurt with a chimney at the top. We were served lavosh, hot tea and kafir, a thick sour cream. These were delicious. We also were served kurmiss, a fermented mare's milk. Kurmiss is milked from the mare and placed in goat skin and aged. It has a very powerful sour taste to it. It is very bad manners to refuse an offer of kurmiss which is the Kyrgyz traditional drink.

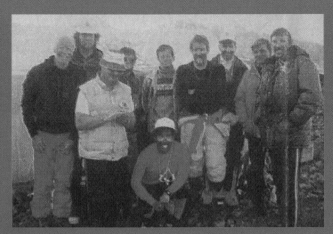

LEMUCCHI (LEFT) WITH SEVERAL RUSSIANS AND
THE MOUNTAIN-CLIMBING GROUP INCLUDING
FOURTH FROM LEFT ALLAN ROPP

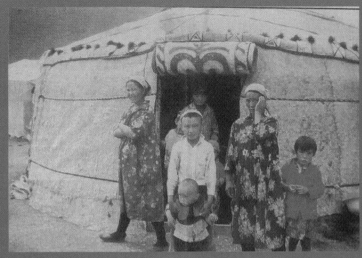

KYRQYSTAN FAMILY AT THEIR YURT

Stacey, Fred, Shasha and I all partook in the kurmiss without showing an external sign of distaste. The patron who was an elderly gentleman was very genial and took a liking to me since I was the oldest of the group and had a white beard.

I gave the patron as well as some of his children some small boxes of California dried raisins and a packet of cookies which were all enthusiastically received. They seemed to enjoy the raisins. We took photos with the family and departed with mutual feelings of good will and friendship.

On Friday, July 29, 1988, we took a long hike down the valley to a lake which was fed by two streams one of which was the Lenin River. The lake was very cold but very clear. Shasha, Fred, Stacey and I made the trip walking in about an hour and a half. We spent a pleasant day swimming in the cold water and sunbathing in the warm sun of the Pamier mountains at around 11,000 to 12,000 feet. Children from a nearby yurt followed us to the lake, and I gave them some raisin packets and cookies which they enjoyed.

After our swim we hiked back past the yurt that we had visited the day before and again were invited in for the traditional repeat of kafir and kurmiss. The lady of the house served us the kafir which was thick, rich and creamy and very tasty. Fortunately, she did not serve us any kurmiss which was just as well since my stomach was somewhat upset from the experience of the kurmiss the day prior. The patron of the house had nine children. I gave him a U.S.A. pin flag with a bear on it which he very much appreciated.

We again left with good feelings, waves and smiles.

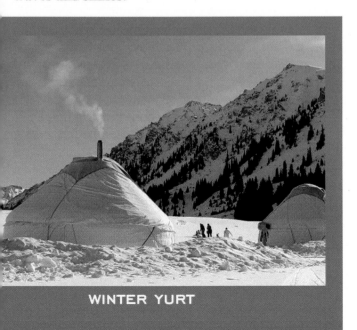

WINTER YURT

peak Communism (from West side)

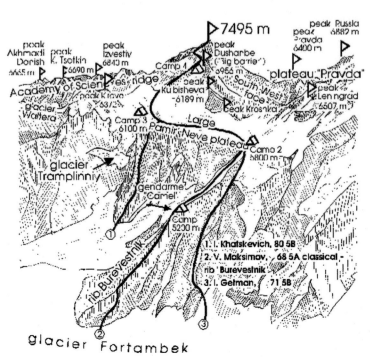

glacier Fortambek

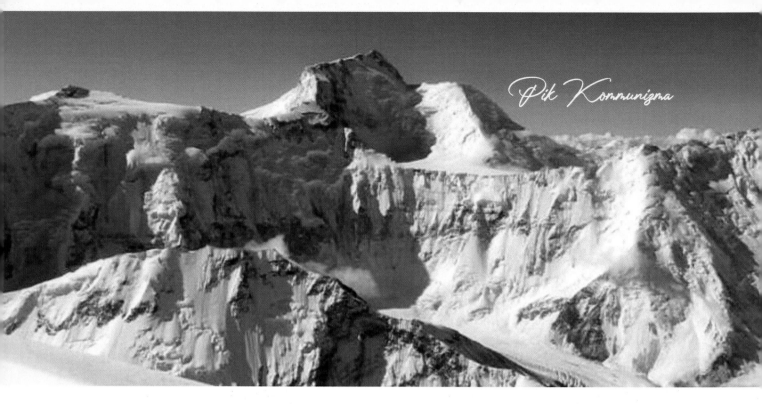

On our return trip to the United States we left Ashik-Tash on Thursday, August 2, 1998, and we were able to stop in Osh where we were allowed to see Allan in the hospital. Allan was still unconscious; his head was shaved and was covered with a purple antibacterial medicine that made him look extraterrestrial. Looking at Allan at that time we all thought that he would not survive. When everyone else left the hospital the main doctors, Stacey and I were left alone. The doctor and his colleague told us in broken Russian what a great nation the U.S.A. was especially our basketball leagues. He was especially enamored with the Chicago Bulls and of course Michael Jordan.

After we returned to the U.S.A. we heard that Allan Ropp's parents had contacted a company called Global Express. Allan had an American Express card and prior to his trip had purchased travel insurance. Because of that the parents and the American Embassy were able to contact Global Express, a contractor for American Express, that was able to get permission from the Russians to fly into Osh and pick up Allan. Again this was at the height of the Cold War and it was quite extraordinary for the Russians to allow a foreign jet to fly from London, England across Russia to Osh in Soviet Central Asia and pick up an injured climber. Arrangements were made, and Global Express did transport Allan from Osh to London where he was taken to a major medical center. We later learned that he did have skull fractures and had some surgery to relieve pressure on his brain. We were told he was making good progress as far as his medical injuries. However, he did have a traumatic brain injury and was making slow but good progress as far as his mental capabilities were concerned.

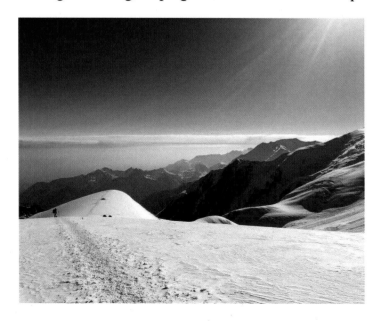

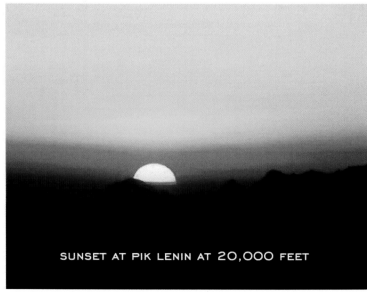

SUNSET AT PIK LENIN AT 20,000 FEET

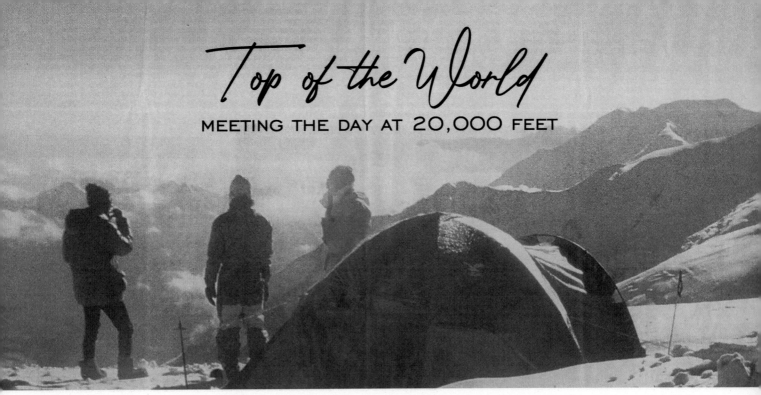

After the trip on September 27, 1988 I was able to talk to Allan Ropp's father in Cincinnati, Ohio. He told me about the trip to London and the surgeries. He indicated that Allan did have traumatic brain injury but was making good progress. Allan's father said that Allan had a great deal of frustration and a short attention span and other obvious traumatic brain injury symptoms but was in good hands with the London medical people and working to regain his functioning. This news came as almost miraculous. After seeing Allan in the Osh hospital with purple antibacterial ointment covering his shaved head and listening to Fred Zeil, an M.D., I thought it was just a matter of a few days or weeks until Allan passed on. Allan made a remarkable recovery.

After leaving Osh we flew back to Moscow where I spent the night and then caught a Finnish flight to Helsinki. In Helsinki I met up with Margaret, my wife, who had just arrived from a trip to Israel. Margaret and I took a ferry from Helsinki to Stockholm, Sweden and then traveled by boat and train to Oslo, Norway. The weather was delightful, and we were in the far north with almost constant daylight. The food was great, the people were friendly and we had a great trip back to the United States. The highest peak in Scandinavia is approximately 4,000 feet and I kept thinking it would not be too hard to make that summit. Maybe I would have better luck in Scandinavia summiting than in Soviet Central Asia.

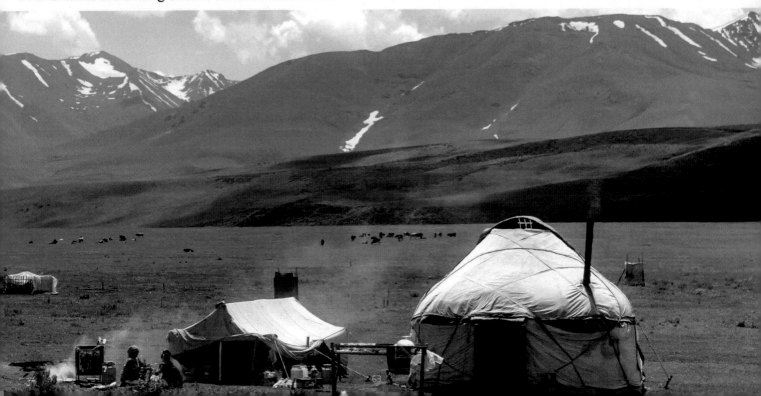

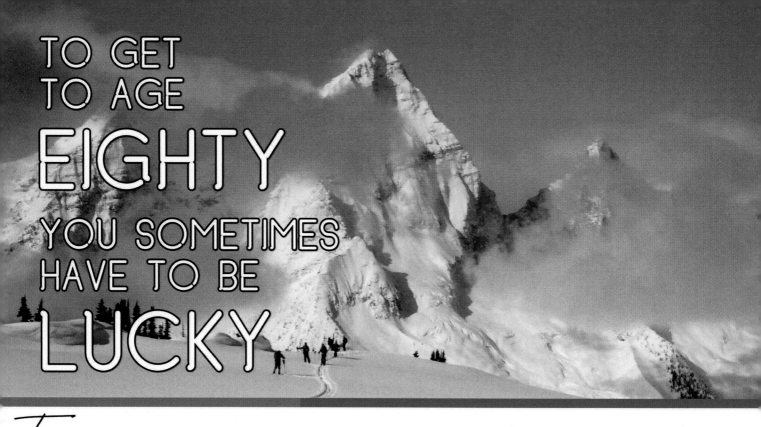

TO GET TO AGE EIGHTY YOU SOMETIMES HAVE TO BE LUCKY

To get to be an octogenarian sometimes you have to be lucky. I was lucky to get beyond my forty-third birthday. Up to age forty-three I lived a healthy somewhat accident, illness and injury free life. But on Super Bowl Sunday, January 20, 1980 at 10:30 a.m. at age forty-three - I found myself hanging upside down in a helicopter that had crashed in the high Sierras sure that my life was ending.

At Mammoth Mountain in January of 1980 where I spent a great deal of time, a new helicopter ski shuttle had just opened and received Federal Aviation Administration permission to operate out of the Mammoth Airport. I was at Mammoth the weekend of January 20, 1980 and on Saturday night, January 19th, I ran into one of the promoters of the new helicopter ski shuttle service at the Pea Soup Anderson bar. Since I was an avid skier I was excited to hear about the new helicopter skiing venture. After some conversation and a couple of beers I was invited to try out the new venture and join the initial ski tour the next day, Sunday, January 20, 1980, which happened to be Super Bowl Sunday.

My plan was to ski with the helicopter group in the morning and then later in the afternoon when the skiing was over return to my condo, shower and get ready to watch the Super Bowl game. I showed up the next morning at the Mammoth Airport around 8:00 a.m. dressed for skiing in full out powder skiing attire: boots, pants, parka, hat, goggles, etc. The company supplied the skis and poles and the skiers provided everything else. After arrival we had a briefing session in the airport lounge where we were provided with snow avalanche beepers in the event of an avalanche. We were told that we would be skiing on White Wing Mountain which is a 10,000 foot mountain just south of the June Mountain ski area between June Mountain and Mammoth. In the summer there is a road into the White Wing area where there is some camping and hiking. The road was named Dead Man's Road because a dead body was found there in the past. The helicopter that sat out on the runway was a brand new Bell 500. We were introduced to the pilot who was a Vietnam veteran with many hours of helicopter flying experience. The helicopter could take four people - the pilot and three passengers. We were told that the plan would be that the helicopter would shuttle three skiers to the top of White Wing and then return to the airport to pick up additional skiers while the three skiers who had been deposited at the top of the mountain would ski down to a meadow area at the base of the mountain and wait there while the helicopter shuttled three more skiers to the top of the mountain and then return to the bottom to pick up the skiers who had skied the mountain and then return them again to the top for another run. We would keep up the process until the guides felt that the conditions did not warrant additional skiing.

Each helicopter trip then had two skiers, pilot and a guide.

I waited at the airport while the first group left for White Wing which was less than twenty miles from the airport. We enjoyed coffee and donuts in the lounge and took up conversation with the other skiers.

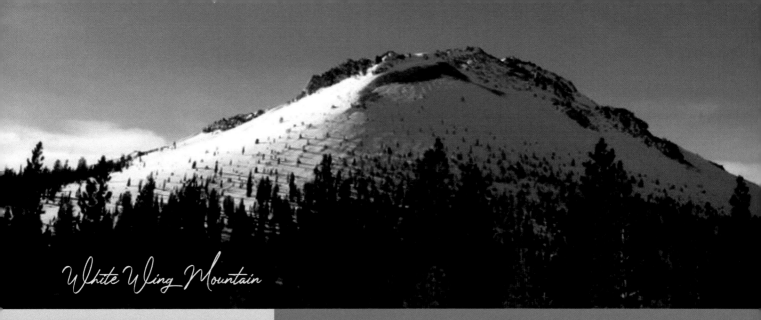

White Wing Mountain

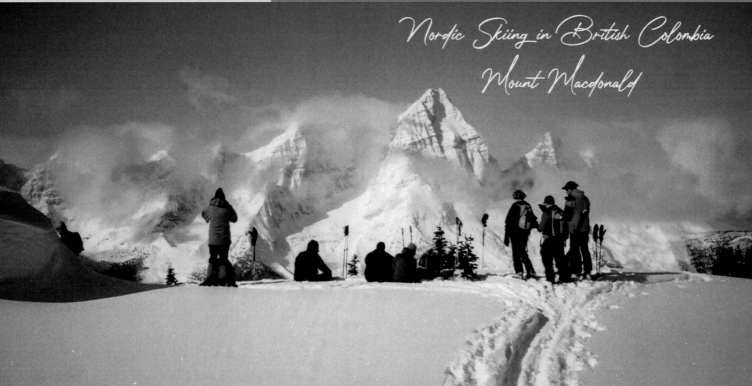

Nordic Skiing in British Colombia
Mount Macdonald

Powder Snow

QUITE POSSIBLY THE BEST SNOW TO SKI. SOFT
AND DEEP, GIVING THE SENSATION OF FLOATING
IN AIR. SOFT WHITE WAVES FLOWING AROUND
THE BODY WITH THE SKIS OUT OF SIGHT FOR
MOST OF THE DAY. THE FINEST LIGHT POWDER
IS OFTEN LIKE SMOKE RISING AND FALLING IN
THE COLD AIR OF A MID WINTER'S DAY. NOT
EASY TO SKI AND REQUIRING A DELICATE TOUCH
AND AWARENESS OF WEIGHTING, UNWEIGHTING,
AND STEERING. WHAT SKIERS DREAM ABOUT
DURING THE LONG SUMMER MONTHS!

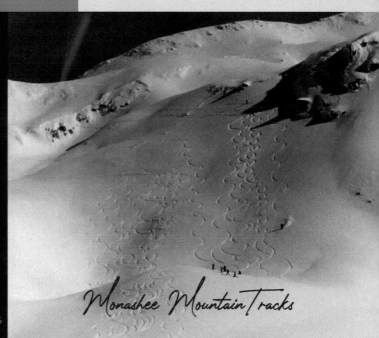

Monashee Mountain Tracks

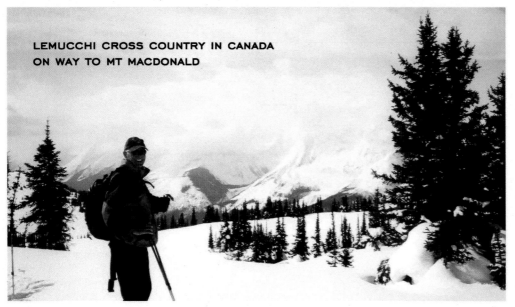

LEMUCCHI CROSS COUNTRY IN CANADA
ON WAY TO MT MACDONALD

Wing where the first skiers would be waiting.

After the pilot left the guide gave us the okay and we followed him down the northeast side of the mountain. The pitch on the mountain was only about twenty degrees and the snow was powdery and soft in the cold morning sunlight which made for excellent skiing. We followed the guide who pretty much stayed next to the tracks that the first group had left down through the beautiful powder.

There were nine of us all together and as indicated the plan was to take two or three skiers to the top of the mountain, leave them there and then the pilot would land at the bott!om of the mountain to retrieve the skiers who had skied the mountain.

When it was my turn to leave the airport we took off and basically followed Highway 395 north of Mammoth up to the Deadman's Road then headed west toward White Wing. It was a beautiful spectacular morning, cold temperature below 10 degrees and bright sun without clouds or wind. The elevation at the Mammoth Airport is approximately 7,000 feet so we only had around 3,000 feet of elevation gain to the top of White Wing. Since White Wing is only a few miles from Dead Man Creek Road the elevation gain to the top of White Wing was gradual and in-perceptible.

We landed on the top of White Wing Mountain without problem. The air was still without breeze and it was a cold and crystal clear day. As we got out of the helicopter we could see where the first group had landed and could see their tracks heading off the northeast corner of the mountain. White Wing is an old volcano cone and has only a few trees penetrating the surface on the northeast side. We had five to seven feet of snow base with a new snowfall just two nights previously. The snow was cold, light and fluffy and promised excellent powder skiing.

We unloaded our skis and poles from an enclosed basket attached to the skid of the helicopter, put on our skis and equipment, activated our avalanche beepers and were ready to ski. Our guide instructed us to follow him down the mountain. He said he would be going slow to start and would stop occasionally for everyone to catch up. The pilot got back in the helicopter, raised up fifty feet or so and then peeled off the westside of the mountain where he would circle down to a snow covered meadow at the bottom of White

In no time at all we neared the bottom of the mountain about a 2,000 foot elevation drop-and slowed down as we skied into the meadow and toward the other skiers who were waiting for the helicopter to return them to the top of the mountain. By now our group was six or seven skiers and guides and were all talking about the excellent conditions and the super ski that we had down the northeast side of the mountain without trees or rocks or other obstacles. Everyone was excited to go back to the top and have another go.

We saw the helicopter coming off the top of White Wing, lifting 50 feet while moving in a westerly direction and then peeling off like a jet plane onto its side and descending down toward the meadow. Someone exclaimed, "Wow, he must have learned that in Vietnam." The helicopter came to stop at a designated spot that had been stamped out by the guides. One of the guides then yelled out, "Who's next?" Even though I had just finished a run I was standing close to the helicopter and someone said, "Go ahead." We loaded three sets of skis and poles into the basket attached to the skids of the helicopter. Once the skis and poles were strapped down and secured the three passengers climbed into the helicopter. The guide got in the front cockpit with the pilot and myself and another skier climbed into the passenger compartment. We had on our ski boots, gloves and headgear. Once we were seatbelted in with lap and shoulder restrains the pilot asked if everyone was ready and he accelerated the main rotor. Again the plan was for the helicopter to take us back to the top of White Wing where we would have another run. As we lifted off from the meadow we rose to an elevation of approximately 100 feet. At that point there was a loud explosion which I later learned was the tail rotor being ripped off of the tail boom of the helicopter by a piece of the engine that had exploded and

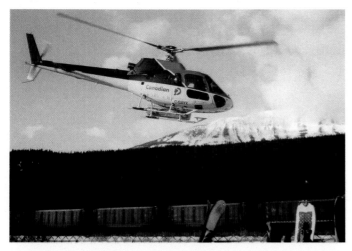

impacted into the tail rotor. The loss of the tail rotor caused the helicopter to start spinning and shaking violently. My first thought was, "Oh my god we are going to crash." Since the noise was deafening you could not hear anything from the pilot or other passengers. It seemed prolonged but actually it was only seconds that the helicopter spun out of control and then fell out of the sky. As we were falling in that instant I was sure that we were all going to be killed. Although it seemed an eternity I am sure that the spinning was just a few seconds until the helicopter fell. We hit the ground with a tremendous impact on one side which I later learned fractured and knocked off the left side landing skid where I was sitting. When the helicopter hit the ground the main rotor was still spinning and the helicopter bounced up into the air, turned over and came back down to the ground upside down with the main rotor still rotating and kicking up an avalanche of snow. As we were falling I knew we were going to be killed, when we crashed and landed upside down I knew again that we were going to be killed. As the rotor continued to turn the helicopter bounced up and down violently because of the continuous turning of the main rotor. After what seemed like forever the main rotor eventually stopped and we were stopped upside down in the helicopter. Again because of the noise we could not hear anyone talking. We were all hanging upside down with our heads down into the top of the cockpit since we were strapped in with lap and shoulder restraints. My first thought when the rotor stopped was that we are going to live. That was brief because within seconds you could hear the engine hissing and gasoline spurting from the engine compartment. "My God," I thought, "we will be burned alive! The thing is going to catch on fire!" I did not know the reactions of the other occupants. I could not hear or see them from my position. I had a terrible time trying to get the seatbelt and shoulder harness unhooked since I was wearing bulky snow gloves and could not really see where the buckles were located since I was hanging upside down like a bat. I was finally able to get my gloves off and then unhook the seat restraints.

That caused me to drop down into the top of the cockpit on my head. I was somewhat disoriented because the rotor had kicked up so much snow it buried the cockpit. I couldn't get the door unlocked so I turned around, lay back on my back and with my ski boots kicked out the plastic door panel and was able to scramble out a hole into the snow. The passenger who was with me in the back came out my side as did the front passenger and the pilot since they could not get the cockpit door open. Gasoline was still spurting from the engine and the pilot was yelling, "Get up the hill. Get away." I scrambled up the side of the hill away from the helicopter and sat back and took a big breath finding it hard to believe that we were not killed. Fortunately the helicopter did not catch fire.

The guides had telephoned back with their radio telephones to the airport telling the company that we had crashed and that we would need to be rescued.

We were told that the plan was another helicopter would come in and shuttle us back to the airport. I told the guides that I was not getting into another helicopter and that I would ski back to Mammoth. They said you can't do that, it's more than twenty miles and there are mountains in between. I said in my state of mind that I didn't care and that I would take my time but that I was not going to get into another helicopter.

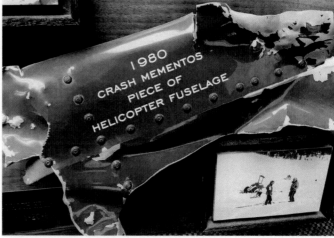

1980
CRASH MEMENTOS
PIECE OF
HELICOPTER FUSELAGE

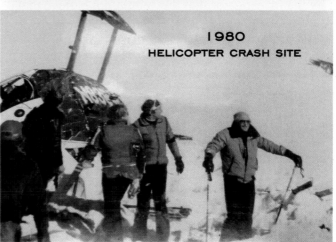

1980
HELICOPTER CRASH SITE

A helicopter did arrive at the scene and began to shuttle the skiers back to the airport. I waited for the last helicopter before I would get into the cabin. The guides did a lot of persuasion but were finally able to convince me to get into the helicopter. When we took off I was positive that were going to crash again and every little movement and creak and noise from the helicopter caused me to panic and think we were ready to crash. I flew back to the airport in a state of repressed terror.

We did learn in taking the helicopter back that if the helicopter that I crashed in had gone another 200 yards east before falling out of the sky we would have crashed into a rocky canyon which more than likely would have caused a fire or more extensive damage to the helicopter and more chance of extensive injury to the occupants.

When I got back to the airport I took my car and left immediately back to the condo. When I walked into the door I sat on the couch and was shaking uncontrollably more than likely from the symptoms of post-traumatic stress. I did show up at my cousin's condominium and told him what happened. During the rendition of the events I did start shaking and crying because I was so emotionally distraught from the experience.

I did not really feel like watching the Super Bowl, returned to my condo, had a couple of beers and went to bed.

After the FAA investigated our crash we learned that the new Bell 500 helicopter had an engine malfunction, exploded and a piece of the engine hit the tail rotor, disabling it and causing the helicopter to go out of control. I did sprain my neck and back in the crash but other then the PTSD had no other injuries. We were fortunate to have crashed in newly fallen snow which down at the meadow was around 10 feet deep which softened the impact of the crash. If we had crashed just east of the meadow in the rocky canyon it would have been an entirely different story. I was also told by the investigator that they could not believe that I was able to kick out the plastic door with my boots since it must have taken super human strength. I responded that when you think you're going to be burned up in a fire you can summon up strength from unknown sources.

Sometimes you just have to be lucky to get to age eighty. Not too many people have walked away from an upside down helicopter crash.

After my helicopter crash one would think that I would not want to take another helicopter into the high mountains.

Well, as time moves on in December of 2004 with my friend Paul Rudder we did a four day Ruby Mountain helicopter tour. The Ruby Mountains arise out of the Nevada desert near Elko, Nevada. The Rubies, known as "Nevada's Yosemite," have peaks of 13,000 feet and have some of the greatest dry powder skiing in the United States. There was some apprehension about riding in a helicopter at first, but after a few dry powder runs everything was fine.

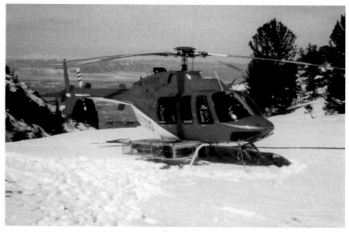

Ruby Mountains Nevada

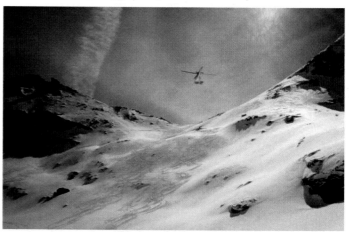

Ruby Mountains Powder Tracks

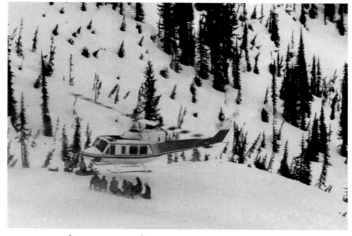

Monashee Mountains British Columbia

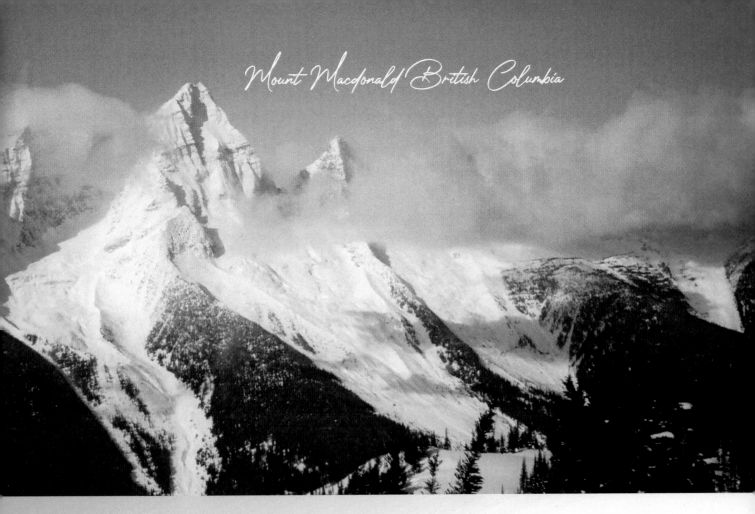

I also have to admit that I did take two helicopter ski tours in the mountains of British Columbia, Canada. These were well-organized helicopter skiing tours in the incredibly beautiful Monashee Mountains. The elevation was around 10,000 feet and the elevation drop was around 2,000 to 2,500 feet in feather-weight powder. There were two helicopter trips to the Monashees.

I also took a nordic or cross-country ski helicopter trip into the Monashee Mountains staying at the Purcell Mountain Lodge on the border of the Selkirk and Monashee Mountain ranges. You access the Purcell Mountain Lodge by helicopter from the town of Golden in British Columbia. The helicopter ride into the mountain lodge allows you to photograph some of the spectacular alpine scenery of Canada's Glacier National Park. The cross-country skiing is particularly spectacular with ski trips to theoverlook of the Rogers Valley across to Mount Macdonald which is one of the most stunning views in British Columbia in the winter all covered with snow and ice.

My trip to the Purcell Lodge in the winter was such a memorable trip that I returned in the summer with my wife, Margaret, to helicopter into the Purcell Lodge and hike the trails through the dense woodlands and open meadows with a profusion of multi-colored wild flowers.

I guess I can say that I put the trauma of the helicopter crash in 1980 behind me with my further adventures in helicopters. In addition to skiing I took helicopters on tours to look for polar bears in Churchill Manitoba Canada and helicopter tours in Hawaii.

... Fortunately none of them compared with the
January 20, 1980
White Wing adventure!

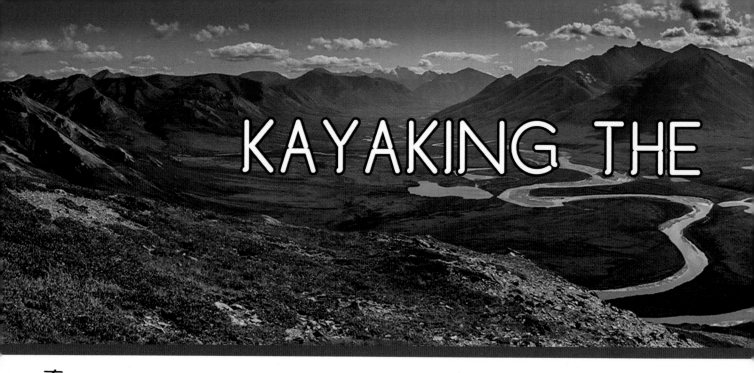

KAYAKING THE

*I*n 1977 I took my family on a 320 mile kayaking trip on the Noatak River in Alaska. My daughter Lisa at the time was age thirteen, Margaret, my wife, age thirty-six and me forty. We had had some previous experience traveling on rivers. Two years before in 1975 we had taken a 90 mile raft trip on the Stikine River in southeast Alaska. We started that trip by flying a float plane into Telegraph, British Columbia, Canada and ended at Wrangell, Alaska on the Pacific Ocean. We had also rafted the Salmon River in Idaho twice so we were not strangers to river trips. We had never, however, kayaked 320 miles down the northernmost river in Alaska. This was going to be something new.

The Noatak River flows through one of the largest undisturbed watersheds of North America basically draining the Brooks Range, the northernmost mountain range in Alaska. It flows through one of the largest undisturbed watersheds of north America and is listed as an international wild and scenic river. The river begins in the Brooks Range in the Endicott and Schwatka Mountains in the Gates of the Arctic National Park. From its beginning it flows in a westerly direction for 300 miles then turns south for another hundred miles into the Noatak National Preserve. The river flows through a wide tundra valley into the Grand Canyon of the Noatak flowing through miles of rolling hills where it eventually flows out into the Chukchi Sea at Kotzebue Sound into the Arctic Ocean. The Noatak River is known as passing through some of the world's finest and best wilderness areas.

It is not easy to get to the Brooks Range and the Noatak River. We started our trip in July 1997 by flying into Anchorage, Alaska then taking the Alaska Railroad train to Fairbanks. The train trip from Anchorage to Denali National Park where we stopped and spent the night is a wonderful ride through the Alaska Range - a spectacular experience in itself. After a night at Denali National Park in the McKinley Hotel we re-boarded the train for the ride into Fairbanks.

At Fairbanks we took a day trip on the Chena River and visited Susan Butcher's home where she raises her Alaskan sled dogs. Butcher has won the Iditarod sled dog race in Alaska four times.

The next day we boarded a small commuter plane that took us into Bettles, Alaska where we met our guide David Ketcher, the owner of the Bettles Trading Post/Sourdough Outfitters, the only business in town. At the Bettles landing strip one is greeted by a large sign that tells you that you are thirty-five miles north of the arctic circle, that the population is 51 and the lowest recorded temperature was in 1975 at 70 degrees below 0 and the highest temperature in July 1955 at 92 degrees. The biggest snowfall had been 116 inches and the average rainfall 21 inches.

Our guide David Ketcher happened to be from Exeter, California so as San Joaquin Valley residents we had a lot in common to talk about. David, his wife and son ran the trading post and guide service. David was going to be our sole guide for the next three weeks. We spent the night in Bettles at the trading post and enjoyed a hearty

NOATAK RIVER
Alaska

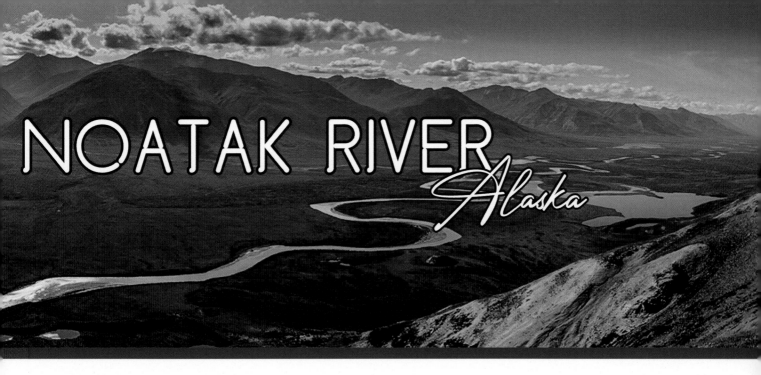

meal cooked by his wife Tammy. A few years later I would be using their son Brandon as a guide on a dogsled trip. The Ketchers were raising Alaskan sled dogs and had some pups which Lisa enjoyed playing with, particularly one named "Foxy."

The Ketchers were interesting people. David and Tammy were working on David's family's farm in Exceter in the central San Joaquin Valley, and after years of farming he and Tammy and son Brandon decided on a new adventure owning a trading post in Bettles, Alaska - a place as remote as one could find from the San Joaquin Valley. The Ketchers had established interesting relationships with the native people who populated the area and sold a variety of goods and service to the native population. David and Tammy regaled us with tales about these fascinating relationships. David's trading post had many furs - fox, lynx, wolf, coyote - which were trapped by the native people and often used to trade for food and goods. I hope one of the Ketchers will write a book about their adventures and relationships with the native people. Over the years I took several trips out of Sourdough with David and Brandon in both summer and winter. Some of those trips are described herein.

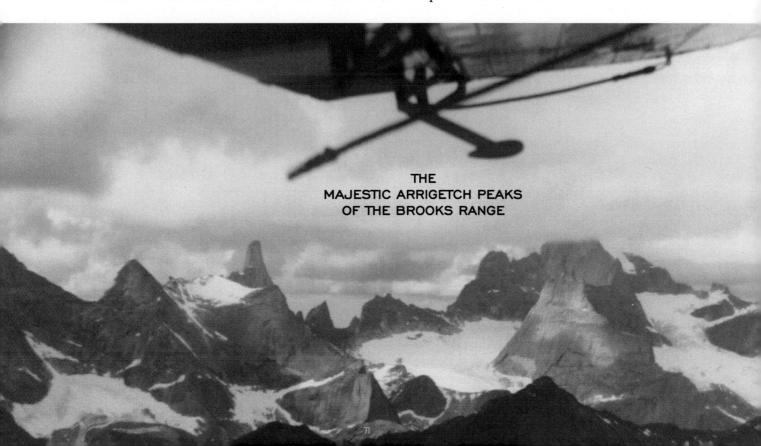

THE
MAJESTIC ARRIGETCH PEAKS
OF THE BROOKS RANGE

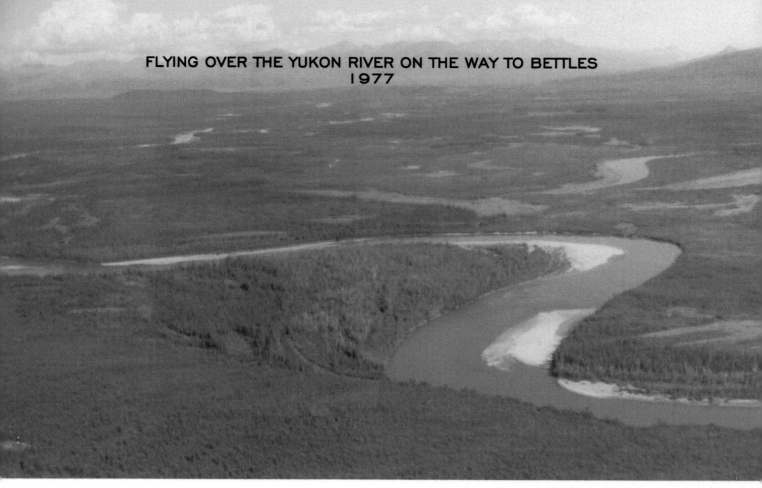

David had assembled all the goods and equipment that we would need for our three week trip on the Noatak. The next day after a hearty breakfast we helped David, his son and his helper compact all of our equipment into duffle bags that could be loaded into our kayaks. Ketcher had a small floating dock on the Koyukuk River where a float plane could be tied up for loading the equipment. David had chartered a de Havilland Beaver, the classic Alaska bush plane, to fly us into the headwaters of the Noatak River. We were going to use collapsible kayaks for our kayaking trip to carry our sleeping bags, tents, food, all of our camping gear and us for the three week trip.

We were planning to use the Folbot collapsible kayaks for our trip. Folbot is an interesting company that started in London, England in 1933 and has a sterling reputation for building a sturdy and stable kayak. The Folbot and the Klepper kayak, a German-made kayak, were the most used backcountry kayaks until Japanese and Chinese versions of the collapsible kayaks came along. Folbot advertises that it takes only three minutes to set the boat up. It is made from double-layered polypropylene material and folds out of a small box. Compacted it weighs only twenty-six pounds. The three minute setup is only for those who know what they are doing - for the uninitiated the Folbot is a Rubik's cube.

The flight into the headwaters of the Noatak was as breathtaking and spectacular as one could imagine.

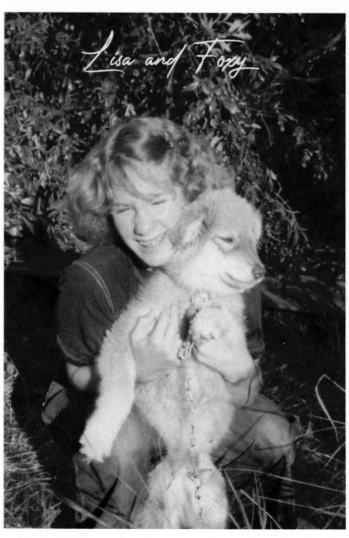

Lisa and Foxy

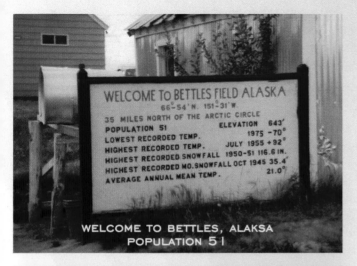

WELCOME TO BETTLES, ALAKSA
POPULATION 51

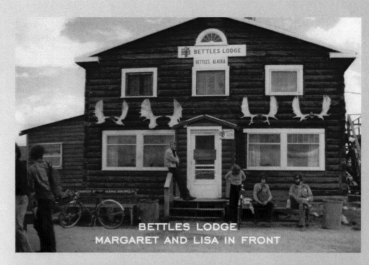

BETTLES LODGE
MARGARET AND LISA IN FRONT

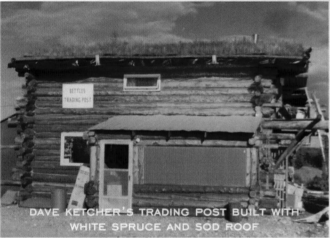

DAVE KETCHER'S TRADING POST BUILT WITH
WHITE SPRUCE AND SOD ROOF

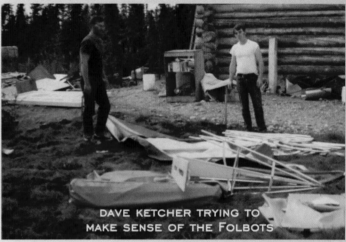

DAVE KETCHER TRYING TO
MAKE SENSE OF THE FOLBOTS

Flying through the Brooks Range over the Arrigetch Peaks is an amazing experience. The flight was about two hours from Bettles into our landing spot, a water slough called Twelve Mile Slough. The flight was truly dramatic over the 8,000 foot Mount Igikpak. After landing we had to carry all of our gear from the plane to the river edge, approximately 200 yards across tundra to a beach where we could start to assemble our Folbots. Good thing we were young and healthy.

The Folbots I likened almost to a jigsaw puzzle. Of course there are simple directions as to what goes where, but thank goodness David Ketcher had performed the task before and was able to expertly guide us through the intricate assembling of the boats. By the time we had unloaded the plane and portaged all our gear to the river edge and assembled and packed the Folbots it was late in the day.

We decided to put in some miles on the river. As our bush plane took off on Twelve Mile Slough to begin its return to Bettles. I thought to myself as the plane faded away - here we are all alone without any of the safety nets of civilization: electricity, medical help, telephone or really any way to communicate with the outside world. I had to think about that for a minute or two. We had about 320 miles of river travel before we would be in touch with the outside world.

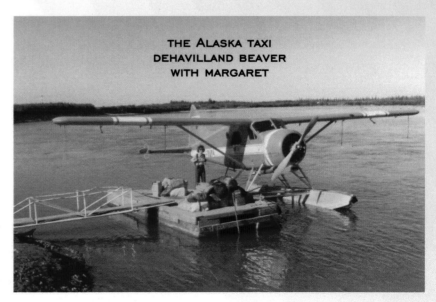

THE ALASKA TAXI
DEHAVILLAND BEAVER
WITH MARGARET

After packing the Folbots with our gear we pushed off and started down the river and put in some miles until such time when David decided it was time to look for a camp.

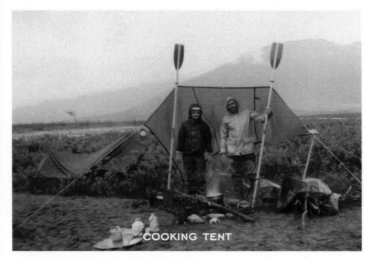

COOKING TENT

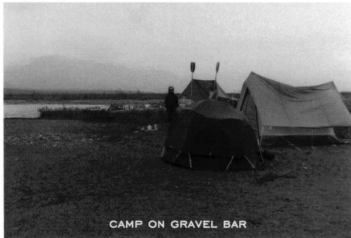

CAMP ON GRAVEL BAR

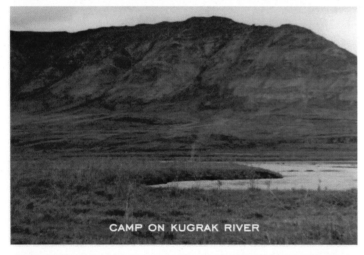

CAMP ON KUGRAK RIVER

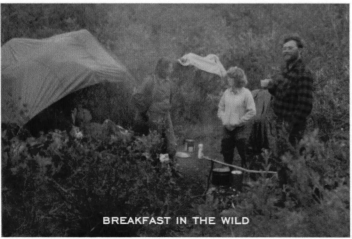

BREAKFAST IN THE WILD

Our first camp we called "Mosquito Hollow" because of the hordes of mosquitoes that attacked us once we exited the kayaks. On the river with a breeze the mosquitos did not bother us, but when we hit land they attacked in force.

We did have mosquito netting and repellant which helped a lot. We set up our camp with a cook tent with smaller tents for Lisa and David. Margaret and I had a Northface tent in which one could almost stand with head and shoulders slightly bent. The front flaps of the tents were all equipped with mosquito netting - otherwise you could not tolerate the vicious mosquitoes. The tundra is their ideal habitat in the summer - water everywhere, warm air and no enemies until freeze-up in the winter.

David cooked our first meal of hydrated stew which we ate in cups as we walked briskly down the beach into the wind so that the mosquitoes would blow away from us as we tried to consume our food without eating extra protein of mosquito flesh. We wore our mosquito netting and would pull it up nose-high to take a bite then quickly pull it back down before the mosquitos could attack our faces. At the first camp I found signs of caribou having come through the area leaving their discarded antlers on the beach. The next morning, I caught several graylings in a sidestream that came into the Noatak. The grayling were twelve to fourteen inches and made an excellent breakfast rolled in cornmeal and fried on David's wood fire. Our initial destination was Lake Matcharak which David said was known for its great lake trout fishing. We actually spent a third night at Lake Matcharak where both Lisa and I caught some beautiful twenty inch-plus trout with bright golden flesh which made delicious eating when filleted and fried.

The course of the trip was quite leisurely, and we pretty much let the river current guide us and only paddled to stay in the main current. We were in no hurry to get to any camp by a certain time. In July in the arctic it is daylight mostly twenty-four hours - the sun only disappearing beneath the horizon around 2:00 or 3:00 in the morning. The Eskimos call the summer months in Alaska "upside down time." No one is in a hurry to do anything since it never gets dark.

Our fourth night we camped on a sandspit close to the water as that location was usually best as there was usually a breeze to blow away the mosquitoes. A mother ptarmigan and her chicks visited our camp without any fear of humans. We noted that all the animals in the vicinity did not seem to have any fear of human beings particularly the little red foxes who came around our camp frequently to stare at us curiously. As we proceeded down the river we would see caribou on the banks, some of them with quite magnificent antlers. We occasionally saw them swimming across the river.

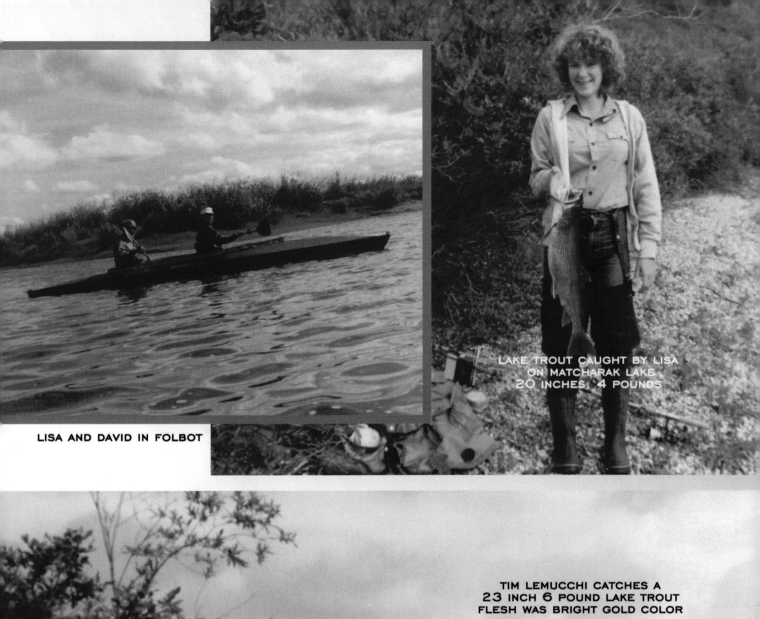

LISA AND DAVID IN FOLBOT

LAKE TROUT CAUGHT BY LISA
ON MATCHARAK LAKE
20 INCHES, 4 POUNDS

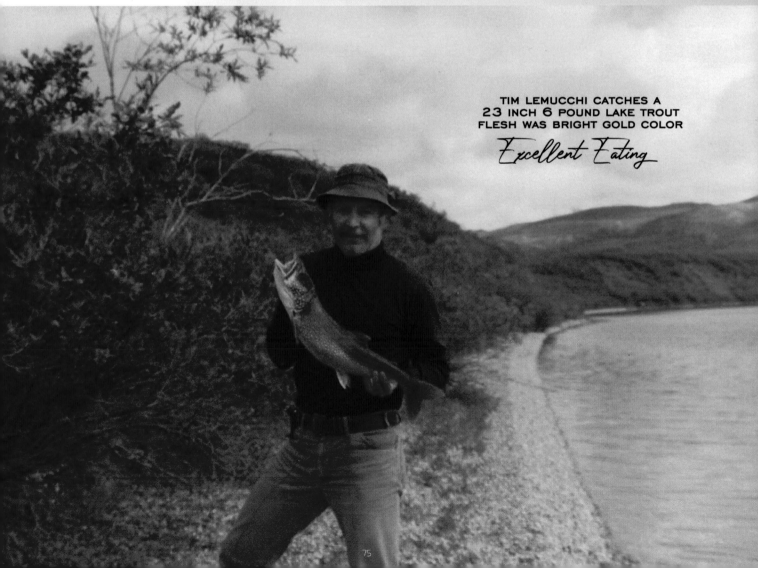

TIM LEMUCCHI CATCHES A
23 INCH 6 POUND LAKE TROUT
FLESH WAS BRIGHT GOLD COLOR

Excellent Eating

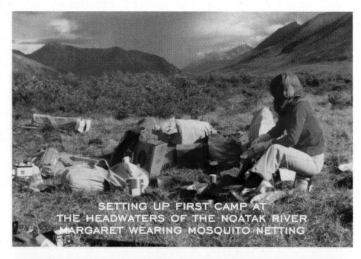

SETTING UP FIRST CAMP AT
THE HEADWATERS OF THE NOATAK RIVER
MARGARET WEARING MOSQUITO NETTING

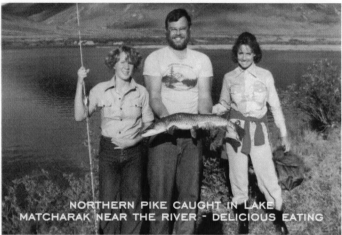

NORTHERN PIKE CAUGHT IN LAKE
MATCHARAK NEAR THE RIVER - DELICIOUS EATING

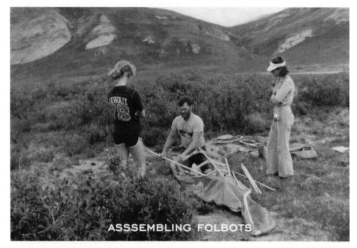

ASSSEMBLING FOLBOTS

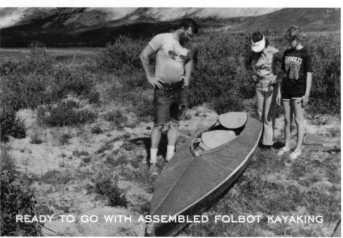

READY TO GO WITH ASSEMBLED FOLBOT KAYAKING

One of the most exciting sights was the wolves. A large black wolf walking along the river bank spotted us and stared at us with great curiosity, and as we paddled past him down the river he started howling and trotted the bank continuing to look at us and wondering who these creatures were. We also saw a musk ox that looked like something out of prehistoric times. At one of our camps we were visited by a porcupine, an interesting creature.

On the Nimiuktuk River, a tributary of the Noatak, a herd of caribou swam across the river in front of us which was quite a sight. We had to paddle briskly to avoid a collision. We usually camped on sandy or rocky spits on the banks of the river where we could get away from the mosquitos. The red foxes often visited our camp, and that night one walked into Lisa's tent and starred at her for quite a while. We also marveled at the arctic tern, a beautiful bird that flies to the arctic in the summer for nesting and raising of chicks and then flies to the antarctic - some 10,000 miles away for the winter season, summer there.

The fishing was fantastic, and each cast would usually retrieve a fish. We also had a minor salmon run where we caught some salmon, filleted them and had good eating. One of the recipes that David used was to fry the fish filets, then break up the flesh in instant rice with some added olives and spices. It was very tasty, and we would often have that. With the daily fresh fish as a complement to the dehydrated food we actually ate quite well on the trip. David's rice and fish recipe is one that we continue to use today.

At a place called Kelly Bar, a long rocky sandbar in the middle of the river, we ran into an eccentric elderly backwoodsman who was gold panning. He had flown his rickety plane from Kotzebue with oversized tires to allow him to land on the gravel strips. He said he was "weathered in" and had been stranded on the sandbar for a few days due to rain and fog. He was excited to see another human being and was anxious to have some human communication. I noted that he had a bullet hole in the tail of his plane, and I asked him about it. He said that a bear chased him around the plane. He pulled out his gun and took a shot at the bear and missed and hit the tail of his plane. He was quite a character. He said he came to Kelly Bar to pan for gold. He had a large water bottle filled with beans he said was his "food supply." He said he pours the beans out of the jar and cooks them for eating as needed. He said keeping the beans in a jar protects his food supply from the bears. Amazingly we saw him again in Kotzebue after the kayak trip had ended. He had flown his plane from the gravel strip at Kelly Bar to Kotzebue and was at the airport where we were catching our plane at the end of the trip to return to Anchorage.

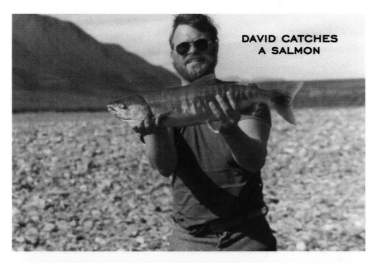

DAVID CATCHES A SALMON

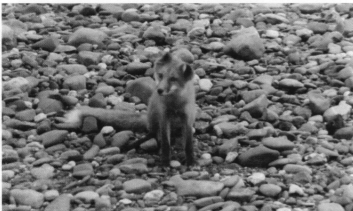

THIS YOUNG FOX GIVES US A VERY QUIZZICAL LOOK, VERY CURIOUS ABOUT THESE "HUMANS"

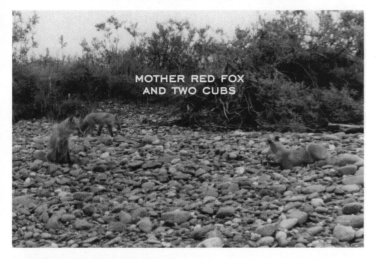

MOTHER RED FOX AND TWO CUBS

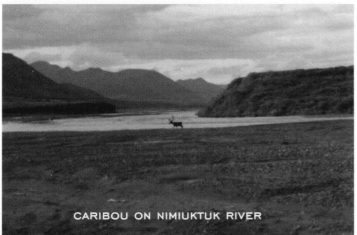

CARIBOU ON NIMIUKTUK RIVER

We departed the Gates of the Arctic National Park and Preserve and then traveled through the Noatak Canyon of the Noatak River, approximately a 70 mile stretch of deep cliffs and some class two rapids which we fairly easily traversed. From Matcharak Lake to the Noatak Grand Canyon we had covered approximately 300 miles of river.

We stopped for a day at Noatak Village approximately 55 miles from Kotzebue. Noatak Village is an Inupiat Eskimo village. Many of the Eskimo families in the village travel to fish camps at Scheshalik on the Arctic Sea coast during the summer, where they hunt whales and seals. The village was officially established in the 19th century as a fishing and hunting camp, but the native Inupiat Eskimos have inhabited the area for generations. The area's rich resources have enabled the camp to develop into a permanent settlement. The village is primarily accessed by float plane although cargo and mail transportation is available by small boats from Kotzebue. In the wintertime the river is frozen over and transportation is by snow machine or ski plane. David Ketcher was a friend of one of the village elders and we were given a tour of the village and met with some of the inhabitants. They told us about their life on the river - interesting exchange of cultures.

One of my fondest memories of the trip is walking on the tundra banks of the Noatak and picking fresh, low bush blueberries and ruby red cranberries from the tundra fields. The blueberries particularly in late July were at the height of their ripeness and were delicious. The arctic grizzly bears also love them.

Another memory that sticks with me is that Margaret and I celebrated our seventh wedding anniversary on July 25, 1977 on the Noatak River. I had stashed a small bottle of wine in my duffle. After dinner we retreated to the tent and put down the mosquito netting, pulled out our cups and shared a small bottle of wine for our anniversary. At midnight the sun was still sitting on the horizon and the mosquito netting on the tent was blackened with mosquitoes. We fortunately were protected by the netting and enjoyed our wine and saluted our seven years of marriage. That anniversary will never be forgotten, wine toast at midnight in full sun.

One incident that I have to recount could have ended in tragedy but fortunately things worked out. Margaret and I were in our kayak alone about mid-journey. David and Lisa were down the river out of sight. It was raining quite hard. Margaret announced that she had to take a potty break. I looked for a place to pull over to the bank and saw a sandspit next to the bank that looked as if it would be a good place to have her exit the kayak and go up on the bank.

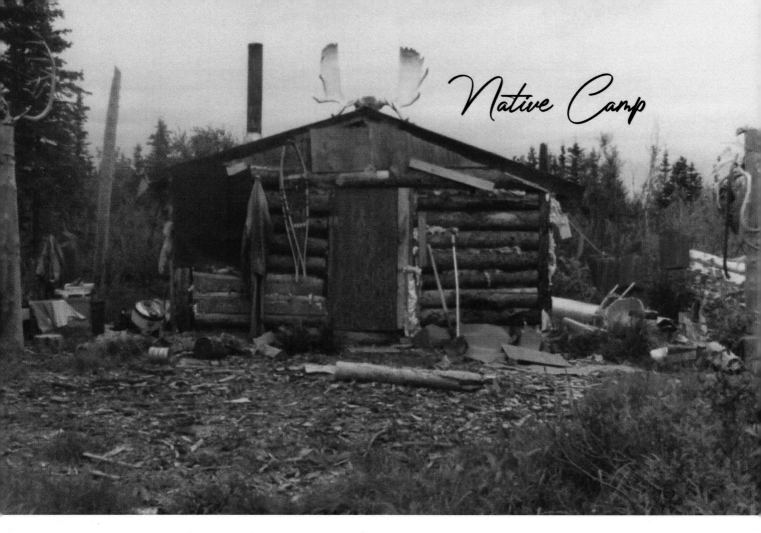

I pulled up to the sandspit, put down the paddle to stabilize the kayak and helped Margaret step over the gunnel onto the sand-spit. As she put her weight on the outside of the kayak she immediately went up to her waist in quicksand and screamed in a panic. She grabbed me and the kayak and attempted to pull herself up which almost capsized the kayak. I had an extremely difficult time holding onto her, trying to stabilize the kayak and trying to move it to the bank. Fortunately, I was able to get the kayak out of the quicksand area over to the solid bank where I was able to pull her up onto the bank. Both of us were soaking wet and freezing as it was cold and raining, and she said forcefully to me, " Why did you bring me on this trip. You know that I don't like this kind of thing. I want to go home!"

I'll end this story by fast-forwarding three months later to a cocktail party in Bakersfield at the home of the president of Cal State University. A guest approached Margaret and said that she had read about our trip kayaking in Alaska (my account) in the Bakersfield paper. The guest asked Margaret, "How was it?" Margaret's response, "Oh it was magnificent. We saw caribou, wolves, bears, all kinds of wildlife, magnificent wild country and had quite an experience. We loved it!"

Bad experiences can fade fast.

The Noatak trip was a unique experience into one of the most wild and scenic parts of Alaska. The remoteness and wildness of the Brooks Range, the northernmost mountain range in Alaska, was in and of itself an uncommon experience. We all carry wonderful memories of that trip.

For me though it was really an opening to the great wonders of Alaska. After that trip in total I have been to Alaska more than fifty times, both in the summer and in the winter. My trips included climbing Denali, dog-sledding through the Gates of the Arctic National Park on three occasions and kayaking and rafting many of the wild rivers of Alaska some of which I will recount herein.

I have always said about Alaska that if I knew what I knew after the Noatak trip and I was just starting out as a young lawyer I would have moved to Anchorage, Alaska and started my law practice there. The access to the wilderness and the many experiences of the wilds of Alaska are unparalleled.

Noatak Eskimo Village

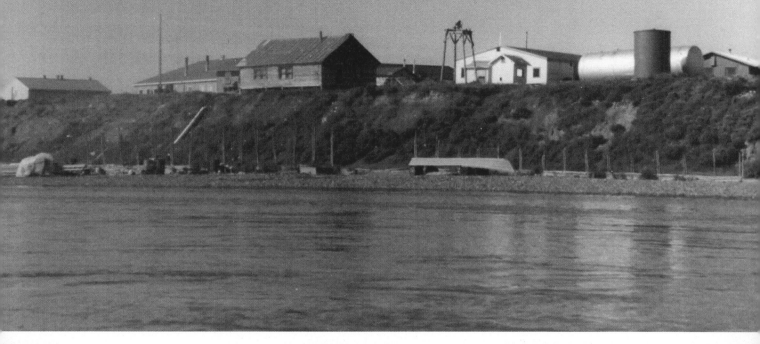

The Great Wonders of Alaska

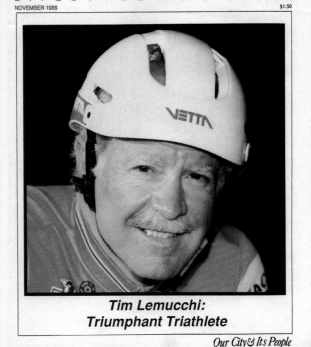

Bakersfield
LIFESTYLE MAGAZINE

NOVEMBER 1986 $1.50

Tim Lemucchi:
Triumphant Triathlete

Our City & Its People

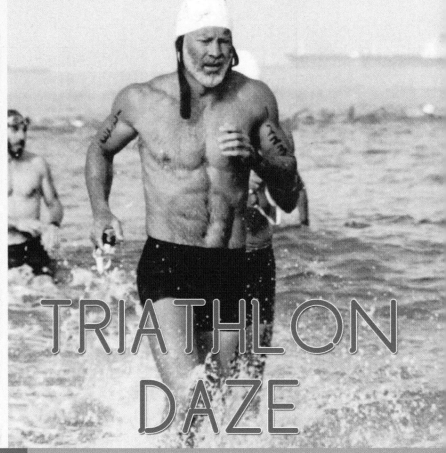

TRIATHLON DAZE

A fifty year old man cannot just get off the couch and spend three weeks climbing to the top and back down of Mt. Denali in Alaska at 20,300 feet, the highest mountain in the North American continent while carrying a 50-60 pound backpack in sub-zero weather. It takes excellent physical health, conditioning, stamina, endurance and strength just to think about such and endeavor. The same can be said about a fifty-one year old man climbing to 21,000 feet in the treacherous mountains of the Russian Pamirs. How do you do it? These are not adventures one undertakes without a plethora of advanced physical preparation.

For me it was just a part of a lifetime of athletics. Fortunately, I was born with some athletic abilities into an athletic family where sports, physical fitness and training were always encouraged. Several members of my family were accomplished athletes and were an inspiration to me to follow an athletic lifestyle.

As a child I always participated in grammar school sports and continued playing in sports in high school and college. I was pretty much an all-around athlete and always played team sports: football, basketball, track and field and baseball. In high school I lettered four years in football and basketball and two years in track and field. At East Bakersfield High School I was the 1954 Golden Gloves Boxing Champion at 164 pounds and in football was an All South Yosemite League team selection.

One of my most memorable sports teams was my first year at East Bakersfield High School on the Dirks light-weight football team. We were undefeated and un-tied and won the league championship beating Bakersfield High, our arch rival, in the final game 35-0 in a game where I scored three touchdowns. I took away from that team a lifetime lesson from our coach Joe Tiner. Joe's philosophy was that you didn't win games because you were better athletes, you won games because you were much tougher than your opponent. Joe trained us very hard, and we were, looking back, the toughest thirteen and fourteen years old kids in the southern San Joaquin Valley. That philosophy of always having a physical and mental toughness and like mindset carried on with me to this day.

My high school Dirks basketball team also won the league championship. Our coach Robert Town really brought out the best athletic qualities in all of us.

When I went on to Stanford University I did play freshman football and junior/varsity football. I also boxed and played rugby, and I was heavily involved in intramural athletics, basketball, football and boxing, boxing in the final intramural championship at 165 pounds.

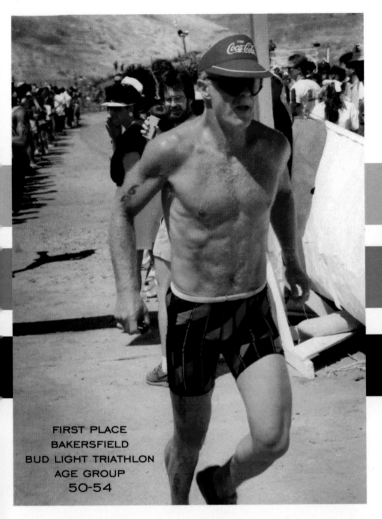

FIRST PLACE
BAKERSFIELD
BUD LIGHT TRIATHLON
AGE GROUP
50-54

HEADING TO FIRST PLACE
SAN FRANCISCO TRIATHLON
AGE GROUP 50-54

After college I did not have much opportunity to engage in sports at Georgetown Law School although I continued my gym workouts and training. After law school when I returned to Bakersfield the jogging craze was starting and my wife, Margaret, was among the first fitness enthusiasts to really take up running. Margaret was a good all-around athlete and was an excellent runner, biker and swimmer. She also competed in and made the championship round of the Kern County Tennis Open Championships. She is the one who really got me into jogging, and with my two cocker spaniels Penny and Peaches leading the way I began jogging a few blocks at a time and eventually those blocks became miles and miles became 10ks and then marathons.

In 1982 I was very impressed that my friend Jim Glinn had competed in the Hawaiian Ironman Triathlon on the Big Island of Hawaii. I thought, "Wow. If Jim can do it so can I." My goal then was to try to qualify for the Ironman.

I slowly got involved in triathlons. I had been doing some serious biking with my doctor friend Ken Jennings and was running with Margaret's encouragement. I was definitely not a swimmer. My first triathlon was at the Costerian Farms Lake south of Bakersfield. The

swimming was in a mud bottom reservoir filled with ducks. We all waded out into the mud bottom reservoir holding onto a rope, a gun was fired and off we went. At the finish of the swim they had assembled a large dressing room where people changed clothes, got on their bikes and completed a 20 mile bike ride through ranch and paved roads south of town. For the bike I loaded up my handlebar basket with apples, oranges, bananas and candy bars thinking I would need extra nourishment to be able to finish a 20 mile bike ride. As it turned out I never touched anything in the food basket as I was so concentrated on riding the bike. I finished with the pack, not a challenge to the good athletes who finished far ahead of me. I was, however, enthusiastic about now being a triathlete. The sport appealed to me because I was an all-around athlete who could run, bike and swim somewhat, a jack of all trades and master of none of three events but could do fairly well in each one. I trained hard the remainder of that year to try to qualify for the Hawaiian Ironman and did so by winning my age group, the forty to forty-five group, at the Bakersfield Budlight Triathlon, the first of three first place age group wins in that event. I worked hard during the summer to build up my swimming.

In October 1983 I was all trained up and flew to Kona, Hawaii where the Ironman is held on the west coast of

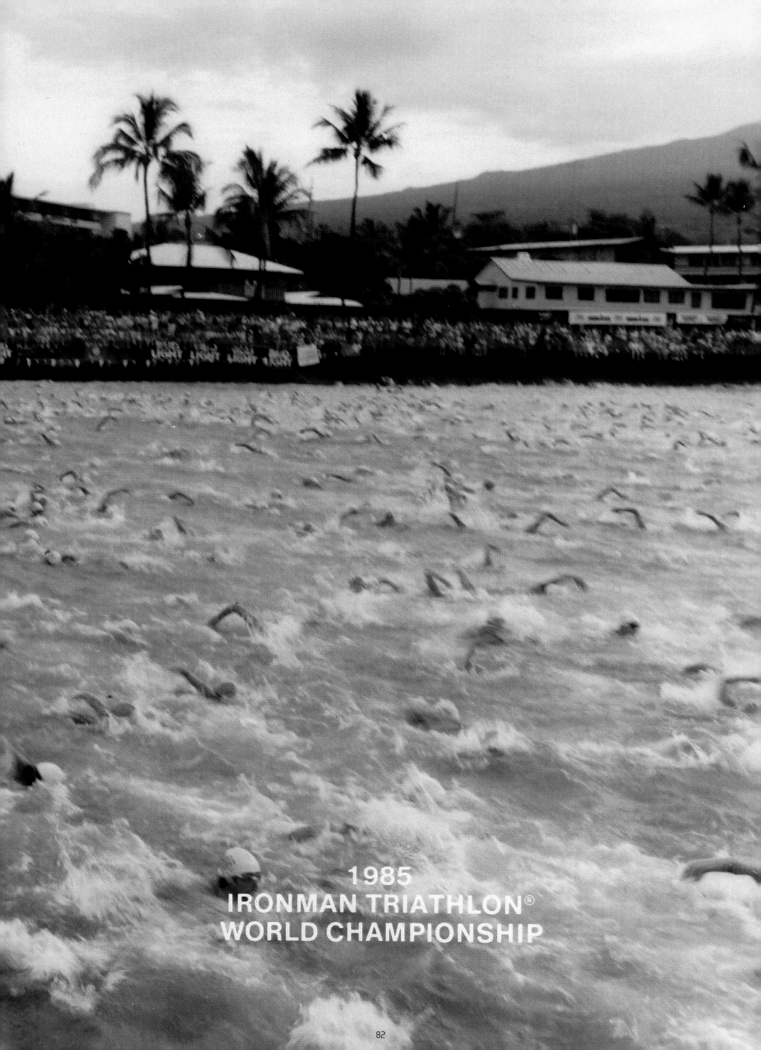

1985
IRONMAN TRIATHLON®
WORLD CHAMPIONSHIP

the Big Island. There were 1,500 contestants and what has always been said about the Ironman is that it's not the distance that is the greatest difficulty but the conditions: the choppy ocean waters, the winds on the bike and the blistering sun on the run. Amazingly I finished fourth in my age group, the forty to forty-five, a very competitive age group, swimming 2.5 miles, biking 112 miles and running 26.2 miles under challenging conditions in under 12 hours. I remember going up to Havii, the small town where the bike race turns around, in fierce winds and seeing a woman triathlete in front me blown over on her bike by the wind.

I was elated after my first Ironman Triathlon, but I told my wife that if I ever talked about wanting to do it again she was to take a gun and shoot me in the head. Nevertheless I did do it three more times thinking that I could finish better than fourth. The best I was able to do again was in 1984 when I finished seventh in my age group which was then forty-five to forty-nine which proved to me that the athletes were getting better and that you had to become almost a fulltime athlete to get into the top 5. That was impossible since I was heavily involved in my law practice at that time and it was my first priority.

In training for triathlons though I remained in top physical condition throughout the year which enabled me not only to complete in triathlons, 10ks, half-marathons and marathons but also to have the strength, endurance and stamina to do endurance cross-county skiing and alpine skiing as well as travel to Alaska for wilderness adventures.

From 1984 to 1990 I was one of the top age group athletes in the United States and in 1984 and 1985 was nominated by Triathlon Magazine to the Triathlon All American team in the age group fifty to fifty-four. In 1986 I won the Los Angeles Triathlon series at Bonelli Park placing first in the master's division in three races with the best combined finish times.

During those years I also won first place in age group competition in the U.S. Bud Light Championship Series in Chicago where there were 5,000 entries; New York; Oregon, 2 times; Phoenix, Arizona, 2 times; Washington; Visalia; Catalina, Atlanta, Georgia 1st Masters; and the Bakersfield Bud Light, three times. Another highlight was a second place in the U.S. National Short Course Bud Light Championships at Bass Lake, California in 1984 and a second place in the National Long Course Championship at Bend, Oregon in 1985which consisted of a 1.5 mile swim and 50 mile bike race and a 13 mile run through the Cascade Mountains at the Mount Baldy Ski Resort in Bend, Oregon.

The training for triathlons gave me the ability to climb Denali, ski the Sierra Crest, ski across the Sierras four times, climb mountains in the Russian Pamirs, take

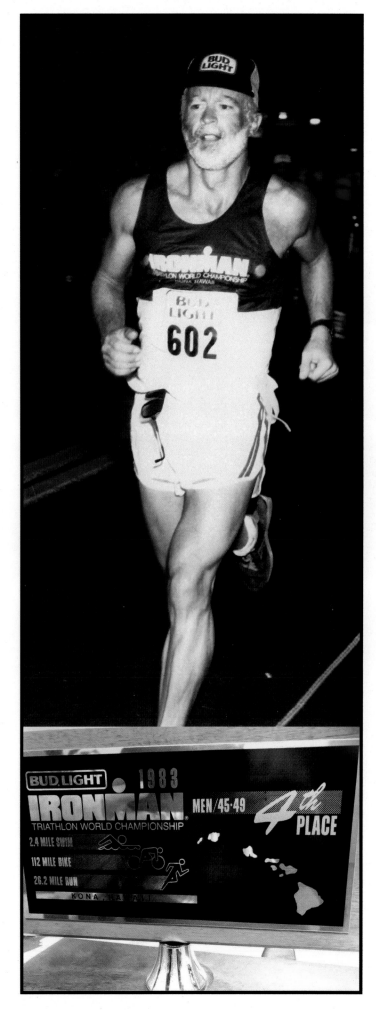

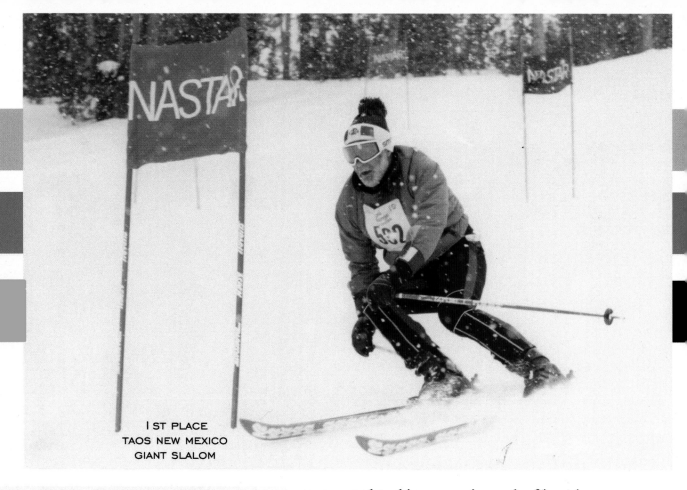

1ST PLACE
TAOS NEW MEXICO
GIANT SLALOM

numerous kayaking, canoeing and rafting trips on Alaskan rivers and engage in many ski mountaineering journeys in the Sierra Nevadas. I also developed my skills as an Alpine skier and won an Open Giant Slalom Race in Aspen and an open Giant Slalom Race in Taos Ski Valley.

I was a consistent Gold Medal Nastar medal winner. While training for the Ironman in which I competed four times I was biking approximately 1,000 miles per month, running 60 miles a month and swimming 18,000 yards or 10 miles a week. My swimming had improved to the point that I was always in the top three of my age group in the swim of a triathlon.

To climb Mt. McKinnley and ski the crests of the Sierras, climb in the Pamirs and engage in other ultra endurance sports it helps to be in superb physical condition. I was able to do these things because I maintained such a high level of conditioning. My training as a triathlete gave me a great deal of flexibility to engage in a lot of wonderful activities.

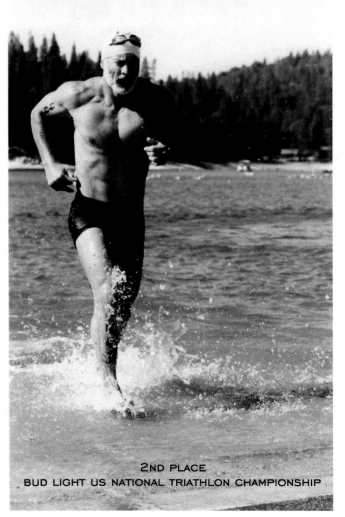

2ND PLACE
BUD LIGHT US NATIONAL TRIATHLON CHAMPIONSHIP

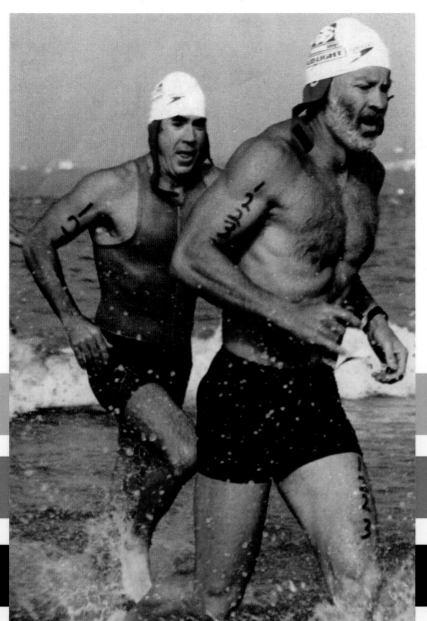

WHILE TRAINING FOR THE
IRONMAN
IN WHICH I COMPETED
FOUR TIMES I WAS:

BIKING
1,000 MILES PER MONTH

RUNNING
60 MILES A MONTH

SWIMMING
3,000 YARDS PER DAY
OR 40 MILES PER MONTH

ALL FOR ONE AND ONE FOR ALL

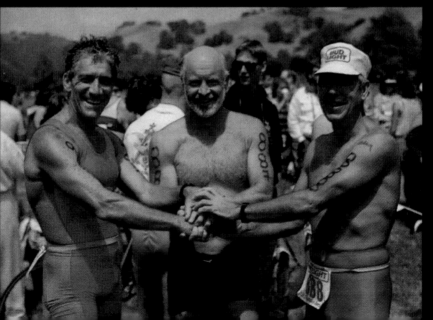

JACK EBERLY

TIM LEMUCCHI

GARY MCCAIN

USTS
SAN FRANCISCO
1985

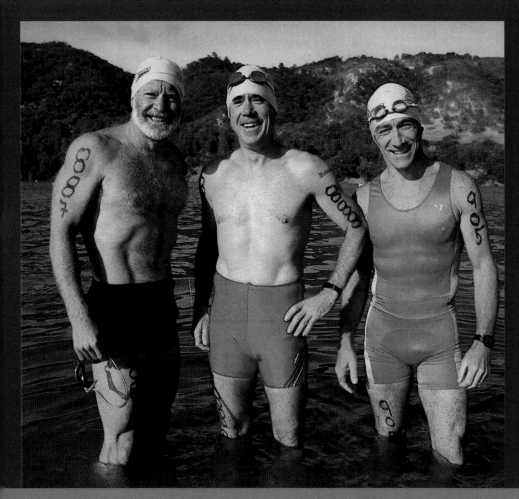

BAKERSFIELD TRIATHLON TRIO

TIM LEMUCCHI

GARY MCCAIN

JACK EBERLY

1987 TRIATHLON TODAY
ALL-AMERICAN
★ TEAM ★

For consistent excellence of performance,

Timothy Lemucchi

has been named to the

1987 Triathlon Today All-American Team

Lew Kidder, Publisher

Bill Zolkowski, Publisher

Jane Gindin, Editor

1988 TRIATHLON TODAY
ALL-AMERICAN
★ TEAM ★

For consistent excellence of performance,

Timothy Lemucchi

has been named to the

1988 Triathlon Today All-American Team

Lew Kidder, Publisher

Bill Zolkowski, Publisher

Jane Gindin, Editor

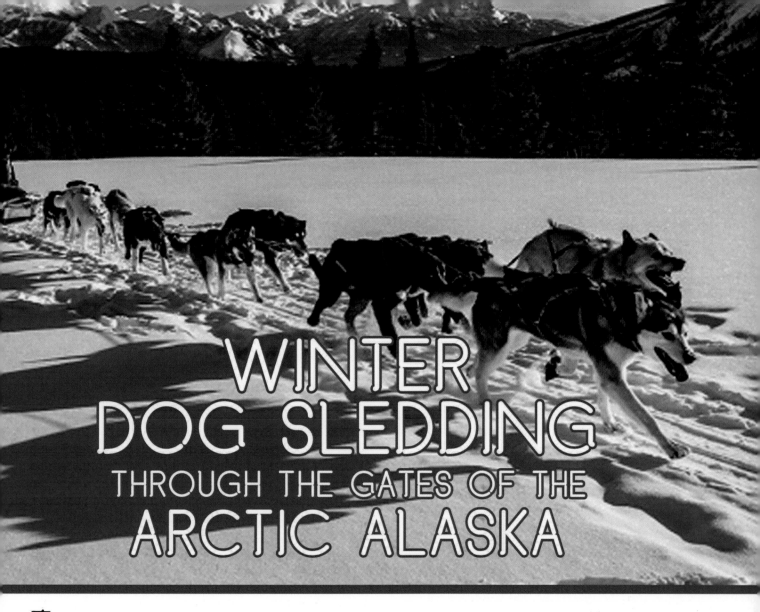

WINTER DOG SLEDDING
THROUGH THE GATES OF THE
ARCTIC ALASKA

*I*n reading my adventure stories about Alaska one can understand how I became so enamored with that part of the world. After climbing Denali, kayaking the Noatak River and rafting and canoeing many of the rivers in Alaska I became intimately familiar with that state and in the course of my adventures there made more than fifty trips to Alaska. As I have stated before knowing what I know now about the great adventure opportunities in that northern land I would have moved to Anchorage, Alaska after receiving my law degree and passing the bar examination to start my legal career there. In Anchorage one could have combined a legal career with the doorstep opportunity to be almost immediately in true Alaska back country and wilderness.

As I became more and more familiar with Alaska and particularly the northern most part of the state above the arctic circle I also became quite interested in dog sledding.

The original seed for the fascination with dog sledding began on the Noatak River trip in 1977 when we stopped in Bettles and had hands-on experiences with Dave Ketcher's hybrid Alaskan sled dogs that he was raising at Sourdough Outfitters. As I mentioned my daughter Lisa was particularly attracted to an Alaskan husky named "Foxy." Since my early trips to Alaska I became fascinated with the Iditarod, the 1200 mile dog sled race from Anchorage to Nome, and would read about the race - the yearly extreme weather conditions, the personal stories of the racers and the profiles of the dogs.

In my conversations with Dave Ketcher in subsequent visits to the trading post he told me that he was raising sled dogs in anticipation of offering sled dog expeditions into the Gates of the Arctic National Park. He told me that he had been talking to Bill Mackey, a legendary name in Alaska dog sledding, about using Mackey as a dog sledding guide and using the sled dogs Mackey was breeding at his home in Wiseman, not far from Bettles.

I told Dave that I was of course interested and to keep me apprised of his efforts to set up dog sledding expeditions.

Well sure enough Dave did put together dog sledding expeditions and when he contacted me in 1990 I told him that I was ready to go. Beginning in February the Alaskan mushers come out of their self-imposed winter hibernation and ready their dogs to sled for the winter season. By February the arctic begins its slow retreat from winter's grip and the sun is well above the horizon and stays up ten minutes longer each day. By mid March the sun is above the horizon twelve hours a day resulting in fourteen or fifteen hours of daylight. This is one of the main reasons the Iditarod race is run in March, it's the height of the mushing season.

As I became more familiar with dog sledding in Alaska I learned that most Alaskans mush dogs say that April to March is, "the best time of the year." Day temperatures range from the teens to the upper twenties although night time temperatures are mostly thirty to forty below zero which keeps the snow in excellent condition.

I had been to the Gates of the Arctic National Park in the summer on our kayaking trip down the Noatak River. I thought, however, what a challenge it would be to go there in the wintertime an experience that few humans have experienced. The vast landscapes of the Gates of the Arctic National Park situated entirely north of the arctic circle extends across a 7.5 million acres and does not contain any roads or trails. Wild rivers meander through glacier-carved valleys, caribou migrate along passes thousands of year old. In the summer the sun does not set and the aurora borealis dominates the night winter skies. The land is virtually unchanged except by the forces of nature. Because of the cold and extreme weather very few people visit the Gates of the Arctic in the winter.

In all I took three dogsled expeditions in Alaska. The first in March 1991, the second in April 1992 and the third in March 1993 all with Bill Mackey and his dogs covering approximately 600 miles by dog sled in the combined trips.

On the first trip that I hooked up with Dave Ketcher I was accompanied by Jim Glinn a founder of the Bakersfield physical therapy provider Glinn and Giordano. Jim was an avid endurance athlete and had completed the Hawaii Ironman and a winter biking race on the Yetna River in Alaska. Also on our trip was Nevada Weir who was to become a famous photo journalist having successfully published books her photographs from Asia, the Himalayas and the American west. She won the Lowell Thomas Best Travel Book award in 1992. Nevada operated out of

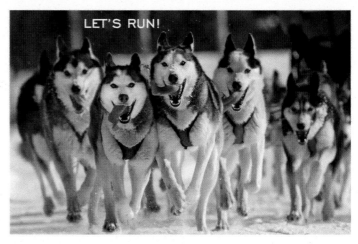

LET'S RUN!

Santa Fe, NM where she had her photography studio.

The third member of our group was Gunter Wehrman, a fluent English speaking German foreign service officer who had come from Germany to experience the Alaskan arctic in the winter.

Before embarking on this trip both Jim and I got ourselves in excellent physical condition as Jim and I planned to do some Nordic skiing as well as snow skiing on the trip and took that extra set of equipment with us. Our small group was to be one of Dave Ketcher's first experience in arctic dog sledding with Cheehako, the Alaskan word for arctic novices.

On Sunday, March 31, 1991 Jim Glinn and I left Bakersfield early in the morning where we caught an Alaskan air flight at 7:30 a.m. from Burbank to Seattle and the on to Anchorage. We had a short layover in Anchorage and took the same plane on to Fairbanks arriving at 4:30 p.m. We were greeted in Fairbanks with news that there had been a record snowfall in Fairbanks and some of the residential roofs in the town had caved in due to the extensive snow. This was a tragedy for the people involved but did bode well for our trip into the Gates of the Arctic National Park as we would have great snow cover.

On Monday, April 1, 1991 after a great steak and wine dinner the prior night at Sophie's Station, Jim Glinn and I boarded a Frontier airlines Fairchild twenty passenger plane for the one hour flight to Bettles. As we flew out of Fairbanks and north over the Yukon River and crossed the arctic circle I was immediately impressed by the vast amount of whiteness that covered the territory. All streams, lakes and the vast amount of greenery and water that one would see in the summer time were now frozen and covered with a white blanket of snow. Wow, I thought, this is going to be a different type of trip. It also looked very cold down there. We crossed the arctic circle at the 67th parallel and started our descent into the village or Bettles situated on the banks of the Koyukuk River. The air strip had been cleared of deep snow but the field was still icy and bumpy. We arrived at Bettles at 10:00 a.m. on a bright, sunny, extremely cold day of 5 degrees. Dave Ketcher was at the airport to meet us and took us on the short drive to the Sourdough Trading Post.

At Sourdough, Jim Glinn and I met up with our companions, Nevada Weir and Gunther Wehrman. We spent the remainder of the day going through our gear. Dave had sent us advance instructions as to what to bring as far as personal gear. This included lots of layered clothing, long underwear, polypropylene long-sleeved jerseys of different weight, gloves and socks. Dave Ketcher would be supplying all other equipment including war surplus boots or "bunny boots" made for the extreme cold and ankle-length fur-lined coats and fur hats for the sledding. Dave, in addition to the sleds and dogs, also provided all the equipment we would need for snow camping: tents, sleeping bags, cooking equipment and equipment to care for the dogs. Dave was to supply all food for humans and the dogs for the length of the trip. Since each sled could carry up to 400 pounds there was no problem with weight.

By 1:00 p.m. we were ready to load all our supplies onto Dave Ketcher's Cessna 180 modified ski plane equipped with skis instead of wheels. We were to be flown from Bettles to our base camp. Even though the field had been cleared of heavy snow Dave's plane was equipped with skis which would aid in taking off on the layer of icy snow that still remained on the runway. The Cessna 180 with pilot Dave, three passengers and all our equipment was fully loaded. We took off northbound toward the Brooks Range and through a low pass into the Koyukuk River Valley, snow blanketing everything. We spot some moose in a creek bed and see a few scattered caribou. We fly up the Koyukuk River to its confluence with the Tinayguk River about 100 miles from Bettles. This area is going to be our base camp, and Dave circles and lowers the Cessna down to land on the snow-covered riverbed. Since this is fairly fresh snow the landing on skis is quite bumpy, but we glide to a smooth stop. Exiting the plane we meet our guide, Bill Mackey, who comes to the plane with a dog team and sled. We unload all our gear into the one sled, and Mackey ferries us and all out equipment to a cabin over on the banks of the Tinayguk River known as the Tinayguk cabin. The river, of course, is frozen over with several feet of snow on top of the river ice.

The Tinayguk cabin is built with spruce logs and has a sod roof. The windows are still bolted shut for the winter as the deep snow is almost up to the roof line. It is dark inside, and we light up the interior with Coleman lanterns. Mackey has 46 dogs waiting for us at the Tinayguk cabin all chained to their tethers. The way that Dave Ketcher had planned the trip was that

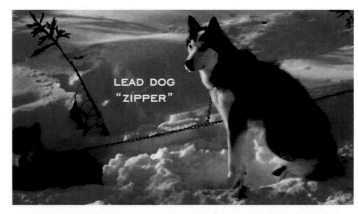

LEAD DOG "ZIPPER"

another party had gone out before us and finished their trip at the Tinayguk cabin and left their dogs there. These people were then flown back to Sourdough in Ketcher's plane. The plan is for us to take over the dogs and the sleds and head up the Tinayguk River then onto the Koyukuk River and into the Gates of the Arctic National Park. That afternoon Mackey told us that we would be taking the dogs out for a run and were to prepare to wear the type of clothing that we would need for dog mushing in the days following. The temperature at the time was below 0.

After unpacking and getting all of our equipment organized in the cabin we hitch up the dogs for the first time for a shakedown run to learn something about mushing. This trip was to be a hands-on trip, and we are to learn how to harness the dogs, know which position in the team the dogs will occupy and how to keep them under control while we are getting ready to take the sleds for a run.

For this occasion we hitched up a team of five dogs per sled just to really learn how to do it and how to mush. To turn left is "haw"; turn right is "gee"; stop is "whoa"; go, of course, is "mush" or "hike" or "go". We set up 20 dogs for the initial run.

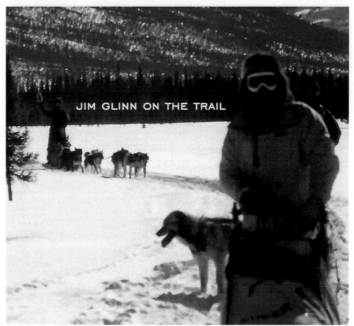

JIM GLINN ON THE TRAIL

We learned immediately that handling a dog team is no easy proposition as these dogs are fast and powerful and take control of the sled immediately regardless of whether the musher thinks otherwise. Also each dog has a mind of its own and is going to do what it wants to do regardless of how loudly you yell out for them to do otherwise.

We learned very rapidly that one must be set and ready to go when the snow brake is released and the dogs take off or the inexperienced musher will find themselves sitting in the snow with an overturned sled bouncing through the trees with dogs out of control.

At the direction of Mackey we get our dogs harnessed and in the correct sequence and attached to the sleds to take a cruise down the Koyukuk River for about five miles, turnaround and head back toward the cabin in the late evening twilight. There is something absolutely breathtaking and stunningly beautiful about the late evening twilight in the arctic. The temperature was 10 degrees below 0. There was some alpenglow, the pinkish glow 10-20 degrees above the horizon, in the western sky. Even through the temperature was 10 degrees below 0 we were dressed in the proper warm clothing and did not notice the cold at all. The ten mile run down and back on the Koyukuk was exhilarating. The dogs were animated and anxious to run, and their athletic exuberance was absorbed by us. There is a unique thrill to running a dog team standing on the runners of a sled in the cold unbelievably beautiful Alaska wilderness.

On the return to the cabin dinner was prepared at 10:00 p.m. - barbequed steak, fresh salad and fresh vegetables all flown in via the Cessna. Since the dogsleds can carry so much weight up to 400 pounds there is no need to bring dehydrated food and we ate extremely well.

At 11:30 a.m. we go outside the cabin to view the northern lights, a spectacular display of eerie extra-terrestrial wavering curtain-like formations dancing across the entire sky in green and redish colors. What a display! This was the first time I had experienced such a vivid show of the northern lights and it was worth the trip just to witness this extraordinary event.

On Tuesday, April 2, 1991 it was 35 below 0 the prior night and is the same this morning. As I indicated the cabin has a sod roof where a bear had attempted to tear into the cabin through the roof and clawed off some of the sod covering. Mackey had to put a tarp over the area where the bear clawed off the sod which was now covered with fresh snow. When the cabin was heated with an interior pot bellied stove the melting snow dripped through the spruce log ceiling and made puddles on the dirt floor of the cabin. Even though it

was below 30 degrees I slept very warm that night in our bulky sleeping bags although my back was against a sheet of ice which had formed on the side of the cabin when the melting snow ran down the side and froze solid. Upon awakening we went outside to greet a brilliant, sunny, crystal-cold, clear day. After a hearty breakfast of eggs, bacon, toast, fresh fruit and hot coffee we began assembling our teams at the direction of Bill Mackey. Every morning was a frenzied rodeo with excited dogs barking and howling all anxious to get on the trail. The crescendo of barking increased as we got closer and closer to departure.

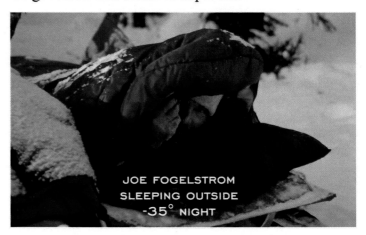

JOE FOGELSTROM
SLEEPING OUTSIDE
-35° NIGHT

Bill Mackey, our guide, comes from a famous mushing family in Alaska. Both his father and his brother have won the Iditarod Race which is a 1,200 mile dogsled race from Anchorage to Nome, Alaska. Bill's father, Dick Mackey, won the race in a photo-finish in 1978, and Bill's brother Rick won it again in 1983. Bill Mackey did the race in 1985. Bill has encyclopedic knowledge of mushing, races and dogs. No one knows Alaskan sled dogs like Mackey. A better guide in the Alaska winter wilderness does not exist.

Bill set up my team with some of his Iditarod dogs consisting of his own special lead dog Zipper, a magnificent golden white husky-mixed breed as a lead dog. In my conversations with Mackey and with his experiences in racing, particularly Iditarod, I learned that the lead dog steers the rest of the team and sets the pace. Qualities for a good lead dog are intelligence, initiative, common sense and the ability to find a trail in bad conditions. A superior lead dog is the key to any successful racing dog team. Susan Butcher, Alaska's many times Iditarod winner, had the most famous lead dog in Alaska - Granite - whom she acknowledged as winning many endurance racers for her.

Next in line for my team after Zipper at lead were Simon and Bomber, the swing dogs. The swing dog can best turn the sled on curves on the trail.

Behind Simon and Bomber came Harvey and Emmet, my wheel dogs just in front of the sled. Wheel dogs are usually the strongest and most powerful dogs.

All my dogs were extremely powerful and fast. My packs and supplies and my body weight totaled up to 320 pounds. I couldn't begin to hold the dogs back. If allowed they would run over everyone in front of us and run at an exhilarating pace. When on the run on a good trail we traveled at approximately fifteen miles per hour.

Our plan on the first day was to mush up the Koyukuk River to a place called Red Star where a tent camp had previously been set up for us. The trail up the Koyukuk to Red Star was excellent. It was a well-packed used trail in the middle of the Koyukuk River. The group that had preceded us had gone up and back so they left a well-packed trail, smooth and fast. The ride was again exhilarating in the crystal clear 5 degree weather.

We did, however, have some funny incidents where one of our mushers lost control of his sleds, tipping over in the soft snow, dumping him onto the snow banks with the dogs pulling the sled ahead. This created a lot of laughs but also a lot of work to get the dogs back in the proper harness and the mushers back on the sleds and on the trail.

It took most of the day to travel to the Red Star Camp. We would stop occasionally to rest the dogs and Mackey would throw each of the them either a frozen fish or a small block of frozen lard, a treat they would wolf down immediately. Both the fish and the lard would give them more fat to burn and more energy.

After arriving at the Red Star Camp we broke down the teams under the direction of Mackey. For each team Mackey would use a gang line section of chain with tie offs. A gang line would be anchored to a tree or a snow stake then strung out usually under trees and each dog is taken off the sled and attached to the gang line at about 7 foot intervals. The 7 foot intervals between the dogs keep them from fighting and eating each other's food. It also keeps the male dogs away from any females that might be in season. After securing the dogs it was time to feed them. A hole was dug in the snow and then filled with freshly cut wood. The trees in the arctic, the arctic spruce, are so dry they would burn almost like paper. We would cut them down, stack them up in the bottom of the snow pit, pour on an accelerate and make a large bonfire to heat water on a grate over the top of the pit. Once the water was hot we would mix it with dried dog food and dish out a bowl of hot food to each dog. As we traveled during the day the dogs would also get their energy treats - half of frozen fish and half a piece of lard.

At Red Star we did not have a cabin but slept in a canvas tent with nets for flooring over the snow. Dinner was prepared on a Coleman gas stove and again was quite filling, pork chops and cowboy potatoes - no dehydrated food here.

Even though I had plenty of warm clothes and a very warm sleeping bag I still slept a little cold that night since we were not really protected from the elements in the canvas tent. The temperature was 35 degrees below 0 that night.

On Wednesday, April 3, 1991 we woke up to a bright crystal clear 35 degree below 0 day. Today is the day we go through the Gates of the Arctic National Park. After waking and having a full course breakfast including hot cakes, sausages and eggs and delicious hot coffee we set up our teams at the direction of Mackey who indicated what sequence the dogs were to be in line in front of the sleds. When the dogs are attached to the sleds there is a mainline cable that runs the length of the team depending upon the number of dogs in the team. Each dog is attached to the mainline cable with a neck strap on one end coming off the mainline that snaps into the dogs collar. When the dogs pull it is mostly in unison.

As we put on the dogs' harnesses, laid out their lines and harnessed the dogs to our sleds the dogs would become more and more eager about departure. The dogs are constantly barking and howling at the top of their voices. They can sense that the sleds are being packed and the team is getting ready to go, and they get more and more excited as we get closer to departure. Since we are now a few days with the dogs they become more friendly and more like pet dogs. They allow us to pet them and rub their heads.

As you load the sled each sled has to be anchored securely or the dogs will take off with it. The best method was to tie the sled to a tree. There is actually a brake on the sled that you can depress with your foot for slowing down or coming to a complete stop. It is not too effective and only works at a very slow speed.

There is another type of brake called an ice hook or an anchor that is used when the team is stopped by either stomping the hook into the hard packed snow or hooking it onto a tree.

Each sled is equiped with handlebars with a crossbar for the musher to hold onto while riding on the sled. The musher's feet are placed on the runners which are the ski-like devices on the bottom of the sled - one on the left and one on the right.

Hands are on the handlebar or crossbar for balance. At very slow speeds and on steep hills it is sometimes best to run along behind the sled holding on to the crossbar or handles to help the dogs with the load. Each sled carries dishes and feeding plates for feeding the dogs and a dipper used for dipping out hot broths and meals. Each sled also carries straw that can be used for the dogs bedding at night, particularly if its unusually cold. Each sled also carries booties for the dogs secured with velcro which are often used when traveling on ice to help prevents cuts to the dogs' paws. Mackey also carries medicine to treat any cuts, bruises or abrasions to the dogs' paws. Mackey also carries a headlight for use in the dark if there is going to be any traveling at night.

All the dogs have a certain "pecking order." Bill Mackey knows the personalities of all of his dogs very well and knows where in the team they should be situated so that they will work well with one another.

Today my team starts with a new lead dog, Rooster, with Harvey and Emmet on the swing and Boomer and Simon, my wheel dogs. We were only taking five dogs today since we are traveling empty to go up to the Gates of the Arctic and then come back and camp again at Red Star. Each of our camps is set up so there is a lead trail into the camp where the dogs can come into a curved funnel-type affair and leave in the same manner. This facilitates setting up the dogs and ending the day. At Red Star Camp it looks like the area where we were camped is set up along an old creek bed which had a bank on each side making it much easier to get the dogs lined up in order.

This morning we have an unusually lively ruckus setting up the dogs. They get more excited as you get closer to leaving with their degree of excitement increasing from the time you harnessed them until you put them on the string with other dogs. The excitement increases into a great shindig with the dogs howling, barking and yelping and making all kinds of strange sounds just before the snow brake is released and the sleds start out for the day. It's like a rodeo coming out of the chute. The lead musher, Mackey, pulls his snow brake and starts his team. When the other dogs see Mackey's sled starting their excitement becomes overwhelming and it is almost impossible to restrain them. They are so strong that they are sometimes able to pull a snow brake right out of the snow. The snow brake is the anchor-like devise pushed deep down into the hard pack snow to attempt to hold the sled and the dogs. Sometimes it works, but sometimes it doesn't. It depends on the strength and the excitement of the dogs. It is best to keep one foot firmly on top of the snow brake until it is time to take off.

There is a great deal of excitement as we leave the camp and head up the north fork of the Koyukuk toward the Gates of the Arctic. A few miles from camp a couple of feet off the trail there is the body of a dead moose calf that had been killed by wolves several days before.

The wolves had been feeding on the remains of the body for a few days, but there was still quite a bit of the animal intact. The cold weather had preserved the carcass and what flesh there was left on the animal. As the dogs passed the carcass they all jumped on it and it was very difficult to get them off of the carcass. The wildness in these dogs really comes out seeing them jump on the carcass.

Several miles up the river we come to a narrow portion of the river where there has been some overflow. Overflow occurs when water seeps up under the frozen ice either by melt by a side stream that comes in and flows over the top of the river ice or by a cracking or pressure so that there is fresh unfrozen water on top of the snow or ice of the river. The location that we arrived at had considerable overflow but had frozen because of the cold weather the night before and it was glare ice. Rooster, my lead dog, freaked out and was completely unable to handle the ice. Once he hit the ice Rooster went onto his stomach, his four legs clawing out frantically trying to regain his balance. He then managed to make it over the left bank where he crawled into the willows and would not come out. Poor Rooster was totally freaked out by the ice. I grabbed him by the harness and pulled him onto the ice and tried to walk ahead pulling him. However, he simply could not master the situation and panicked and headed for the shore. We were unable to get Rooster out of the bushes and had to switch leads. We put Simon on the lead and Rooster back in the team. Simon did a good job on the ice. He was older and more experienced. In a few places we cracked through the ice but it was not very deep, only a few inches, so we did not get too wet. Sometimes overflow can be very deep to several feet and you can easily go up to your knees or hips in cold icy water. Luckily the ice held.

We also came to a few places on the river where there was "rubber ice." Rubber ice is exactly what it sounds like. The ice is thin but not brittle enough to break so when you are on it, undulates just like rubber. The ice is actually floating on the water underneath as the river does not freeze solid. We covered about fifteen miles up the Koyukuk until we arrived at the heart of the Gates of the Arctic. The Gates of the Arctic are named for two peaks - one on the northside of the Koyukuk and one on the southside of the Koyukuk.

On the northside was Frigid Craig, a peak of 5,501 feet and on the southside Boreal Mountain, a peak of 6,654 feet. Boreal is a very impressive jagged peak. Both peaks are covered with snow and ice, and the valley between them forms the entry way to the Gates of the Arctic which is the main geographical feature for which the Gates of the Arctic National Park is named.

We passed through the Gates of the Arctic and traveled up the Koyukuk about as far as we thought we should go with the ice situation and then turned around and headed back to the Red Star Camp.

Bill Mackey has more than seventy dogs at his home in Wiseman that he raises for sled dog use but primarily racing. His dogs are a mixture of Siberian Malamut and Alaskan Husky. He has some black labradors in the mixture. His father, the original Iditarod winner, taught him about interbreeding the black labrador because of their strength and disposition. When the dogs are about seven months to a year old Bill Mackey harnesses them up to sleds in the winter and wagons in the summer to begin their training as pullers and sled dogs. Mackey says that when you first harness the dogs the leaders tend to stand out. Mackey's lead dog, Zipper, was an outstanding dog from the beginning. Mackey says he's been offered more than $1,000.00 for Zipper but is not interested in selling him.

Thursday, April 4, 1991 This was a rest day for the dogs. The temperature was the same, 30 below 0. When we woke in the morning we found that the dogs were all leashed up to their chains with snow that had drifted over them in the night. We put down a little hay for them to lie on but otherwise they sleep out in the cold. The snow blows over them and probably shields them to some extent from the cold. In the morning they stand up, shake off the snow and stretch and wait to be fed.

When running dogs the source of your power is the dogs, and the better you care for them the better they will feel and the better they will perform. Your control of your sled comes from the lead dog who keeps all the other dogs in line. Before pulling your ice hook and taking off you should try to make contact with the lead dog to let him know that you are going to start.

If a dog has been pulling well and you notice that the dog starts to look back a lot, the dog is trying to tell you something is wrong. The dog might need some foot care.

In riding a sled one learns quickly to lean into the corners. If a corner is very tight you might have to get off the runners and run around the corner while holding onto the handle bar. Pumping with one foot really helps the dogs especially going uphill. Running with

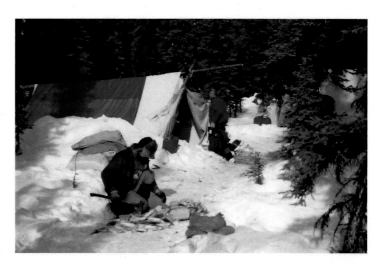

your hands on the crossbars going up steep hills is a big help to the dogs pulling the sled and also great exercise for the musher. Since we were taking a day of rest Jim Glinn, Nevada Weir and I took a side trip. I used my cross country skis and Jim and Nevada traveled on snow shoes with ski poles. We left camp and traveled up over the ridge to Red Star Lake and back - a trip of about five miles which was slow going because the snow was pretty deep.

On Friday, April 5, 1991 it was again very cold - 30 degrees below zero. We got up, packed up our gear but did not get started because of unforseen delays until around 2:30 p.m. Again starting out with five teams is like a rodeo. We struck out going southbound on the Koyukuk River through spectacular scenery again passed Frigid Craig and Boreal Mountain, the twin entrance monuments to the Gates of the Arctic National Park named by the explorer Robert Marshal in 1929. After about an hour on the trail we stopped and fed the dogs half of a frozen white fish. The snack energized the dogs, and again we were off and racing at 15 miles per hour over the dry powdery snow. It was a wonderful ride in 0 degree weather with the bright arctic sun down through the heart of the Brooks Range on the Koyukuk River which Robert Marshal called as beautiful as "a thousand Yosemites." The Koyukuk Valley was ringed with snow- shrouded peaks, and the silence was broken only by the jingle of the harnesses and the squeaking of snow beneath the runners and the panting of the dogs. We raced passed strands of cottonwood, willow and spruce and occasionally routed some caribou and in spite of the temperature it seemed pleasantly warm, and I kept thinking to myself that there is not another place that I would rather be. I doubted that there were any other people in the entire 8.5 million acres of the Gates of the Arctic National Park on Friday, April 5, 1991. I felt very special.

Our camp that night was to be at Peggy's Cabin just below Delay Pass. Peggy's Cabin was of log and sod roof construction but very tight and very warm with a

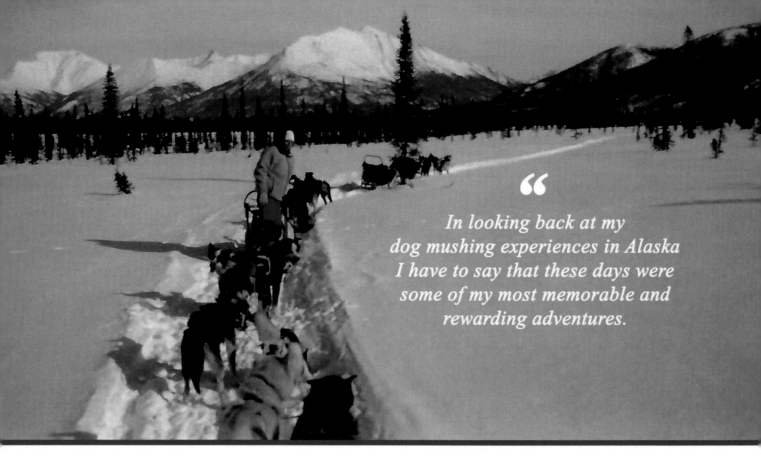

In looking back at my dog mushing experiences in Alaska I have to say that these days were some of my most memorable and rewarding adventures.

nice woodstove interior. There was a very small opening into the cabin that we had to crawl through (designed to keep the bears out and the heat in). The cabin was named for Bill Mackey's sister-in-law and was very cozy once the stove warmed the interior of the cabin. Outside the cabin there was a spring with crystal clear cold water. It was a delight to sample.

After a hearty dinner we roll into our sleeping bags and sleep on a tarp on the dirt floor with our sleeping pads. It was reasonably warm even though it was below 30 degrees outside.

The next morning was 35 degrees below 0. We reluctantly got out of our warm bags and packed out gear, loaded our sleds, lined out our dogs, had a solid breakfast and had another day of rodeo taking off from the cabin. Gunther did not make the first curve and took a spectacular spill with his sled rolling over and his dogs pulling it several hundred yards down the trail with Gunther floating around in the snow trying to get organized.

This morning I was set up with an all-female team of ten dogs. I had a double lead with Emmy and Amy and the incomparable female dog -Jumper- in swing position. What a day I had with these female dogs. In my opinion the females were faster and more durable than the male dogs. My team was very fast in spite of our loads. We went up over Delay Pass with some pedaling and walking at an elevation of 1,500 feet without a problem.

Before leaving the Koyukuk River we traveled through a narrow canyon of glare ice. The female dogs were somewhat skittish but okay. The male dogs did not do as well.

Once we topped out over Delay Pass we exited the Gates of the Arctic National Park and we crossed a frozen lake and ran down Glacier Creek. We were on our way to Wiseman which was Mackey's home and our last stop.

There was another pass we had to go over, Pasco Pass, before we headed down Wiseman Creek, a long narrow canyon with an equally narrow trail with lots of trees. One had to brake often to avoid losing control and going around through the trees. It was an exhilarating fast woop-di-do and thrilling ride. We did not arrive at Mackey's home in Wiseman until 7:30 p.m. where we were greeted by his wife, Katie, and his three children Isaac, Bridget and Becky. Bill and Katie live in a sixty-year old log cabin with their three children and raise over 100 Alaskan sled dogs for racing. They also have 2 cats and a turtle. Bill supplies dogs for the Iditarod, the Coldfoot Classic and the Kanik Races. Katie Mackey is a veterinarian which helps to keep the dogs healthy.

Upon arriving at Mackey's encampment we un-harnessed our dogs, and each dog was hooked up to his own dog house where he had a straw bed and was fed.

After getting the dogs settled we returned to Mackey's log cabin where we had hot drinks and dinner with Mackey and his children. The conversation was about the Iditarod, raising dogs and living in the Alaskan wilderness.

That night we slept in a shack at the rear of the Mackeys' log cabin. There was no electricity in the shack and heat was from an oil drum fire stove which burns spruce logs. After the fire burned awhile the interior of the shack was quite warm and we could move around in short-sleeves.

On Sunday, April 7, 1991 we were up early for a pancake breakfast and hitched up dog teams and took the trail from Wiseman down to Coldfoot which is a truck stop on the Alaska highway that was built by Bill Mackey's father. That January of 1991 Coldfoot had the coldest temperature of 82 below 0. We had a late lunch at the Coldfoot truck stop with some cold beers. We didn't hook up the dogs and start back to Wiseman until about 9:00 p.m. and ran the route back to Wiseman in twilight and dark not arriving until 11:00 p.m. It was a beautiful experience mushing in the arctic night following Mackey with his headlight. The cold was not a problem. When returning to Mackey's log cabin we watched videos of the Iditarod race and went to bed about 12:00 p.m.

On Monday, April 8, 1991 after an omelet breakfast we walked around Wiseman Village. Wiseman was an old mining camp that was made famous by Robert Marshal who spent a year there and wrote a book about his experience called The Arctic Village. Joe Harrington, an Iditarod racer, has Northstar Kennels there in Wiseman and raises racing dogs. He has a wolf attached to a long tether at his property. The wolf has appeared in the movie White Fang. He has some other famous sled dogs, a Siberian mixture, that have appeared in movies as well. After touring Wiseman on foot we returned and packed up our gear to wait for Dave Ketcher who arrived in his ski plane at about 10:00 a.m. and ferried us back to Bettles. There we passed some time at the Trading Post until the 4:30 flight to Fairbanks on Frontier Airlines.

Back in Fairbanks, Jim Glinn and I had a great dinner at Pike's Landing where we recounted all the poignant episodes of our arctic dog sled adventure, both thrilled with the experience.

On Tuesday, April 9, 1991 at 11:40 a.m. Jim and I departed on Alaska Airlines to Anchorage, Seattle and back to Burbank and drove on back to Bakersfield.

My second dog sled trip was the next year about the same time and included Jim Glinn, Gary McCain and Joe Fogelstrom.

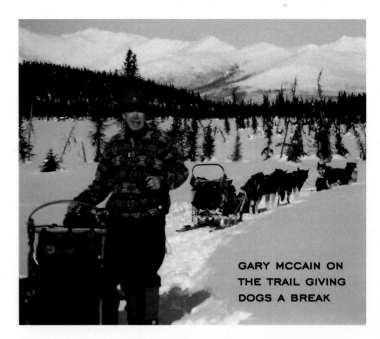

GARY MCCAIN ON THE TRAIL GIVING DOGS A BREAK

We started our trip on April 5, 1992 leaving from Fairbanks on Frontier Flying Service in a small plane directly into Wiseman where we met up with Bill Mackey and Katie. Again we all got a hands-on refresher training course from Bill at Wiseman on how to harness dogs, prepare and to take care of the sleds and feed the dogs. As with the prior trip everyone was expected to help with the chores - gathering firewood, melting snow for water and harnessing and feeding the dogs and similar tasks.

On Sunday, April 5th we left Wiseman on a reverse course and went over Pasco Pass at 1,500 feet down the canyon into the north fork of the Koyukuk River. The climb up to the top of Pasco Pass was somewhat steep and rather slow and required often running behind the sled to help the dogs with the weight. The trip down Pasco Pass was another story. The trail was steep and narrow with lots of turns. With the weight of the sleds the dogs could pull at a fast speed and it was often necessary to keep one's foot on the brake, particularly in going around corners. Gary McCain was behind me with his sled and dogs and I was picking up speed going down through the steep turns where I leaned too far to the right in a left turn, overturned the sled and rolled down the bank. McCain was able to bring his sled to a stop and had a hearty laugh while I climbed back up to the trail. The dogs fortunately had stopped with the overturned sled but it was quite a harrowing experience. We made it to the bottom of Pasco Pass without any trouble, then climbed up over Delay Pass down the other side through the glacier river drainage covering some 50 miles that first day to Red Star Camp. The first night we camped in tents called arctic ovens which when assembled would allow one to stand upright in the tent. The tents were equipped with a small stove that had a stovepipe that exited through a fitting in the roof of the tent. Again the arctic spruce

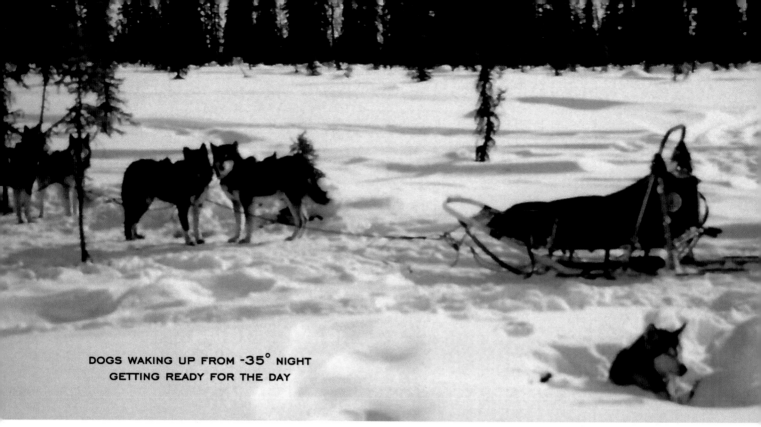

DOGS WAKING UP FROM -35° NIGHT
GETTING READY FOR THE DAY

trees were so dry that we could burn them easily in the small stove which would warm the interior of the tent quite nicely making sleeping at night very comfortable even in 30 to 40 degrees below 0 weather. Again we took good food and ate well on the trip. Mackey supplied all of the tents, equipment, sleeping bags, pads, parkas, bunny boots, insulated mittens, parkas and snow shoes and harnesses.

We traveled up the Koyukuk River again running into overflows and rubber ice. We were all pretty good mushers by this time and moved quite rapidly from April 6th through April 10th up the Koyukuk often running into migrating caribou and occasional moose. We continued up the north fork of the Koyukuk and passed the majestic Mt. Donnerack at 7,457 feet - a spectacular peak covered with snow and ice. Robert Marshal called it the Matterhorn of the Arctic. We paused for awhile on the trail to savor the view and the experience of Mt. Donnerack the epitome of the extreme wilderness and isolation of the arctic North American continent. We headed up Ernie Creek through beautiful isolated snow fields. Ernie Creek was named after Ernie Johnson, a good friend of Robert Marshal, who had a small cabin on the creek in the 1920s. We headed northwest toward Anaktubuk Pass where there was an Eskimo village, our turn-around destination. We camped on Ernie Creek in the arctic tents and slept warm and dry with the spruce trees burning in the small stove. The next day we started back to Wiseman camping two more nights on the return trip the last night at Red Star covering almost 300 miles by dog sled through some of the beyond beautiful Alaska wilderness.

There are those that have criticized dog mushing as being cruel and inhumane to the animals. In my experiences in Alaska with dog mushing nothing can be further from the truth. The mushers love the wilderness, the cold and the excitement of being whisked on top of hard-packed snow at 15 miles per hour by 8 to 10 fur friends who absolutely relish the task that you have assigned to them. The dogs love the outdoors, the human comradery and the opportunity to pull a sled over a wilderness trail.

In looking back at my dog mushing experiences in Alaska I have to say that these days were some of my most memorable and rewarding adventures. Being a committed dog lover and a life long naturalist who loves wilderness in its original unbridled form with no human interferences, dog mushing through the Gates of the Arctic National Park in Alaska is the ultimate outdoor wilderness adventure.

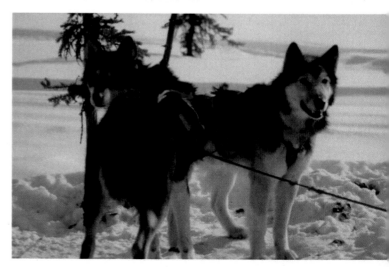

The Gates of the Arctic

IS A MOST IMPRESSIVE SITE PARTICULARLY IN THE ISOLATED WINTER

WE PAUSED FOR AWHILE TO
SAVOR THE VIEW AND THE EXPERIENCE

THE EXTREME WILDERNESS OF THE ARCTIC NORTH AMERICAN CONTINENT

MT. DONNERACK - GATES OF THE ARCTIC

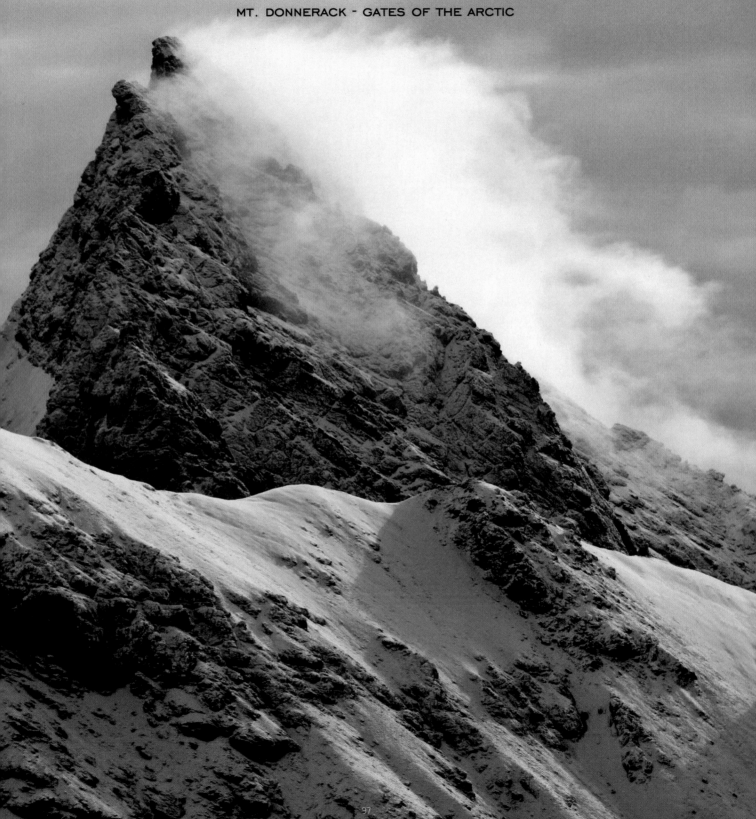

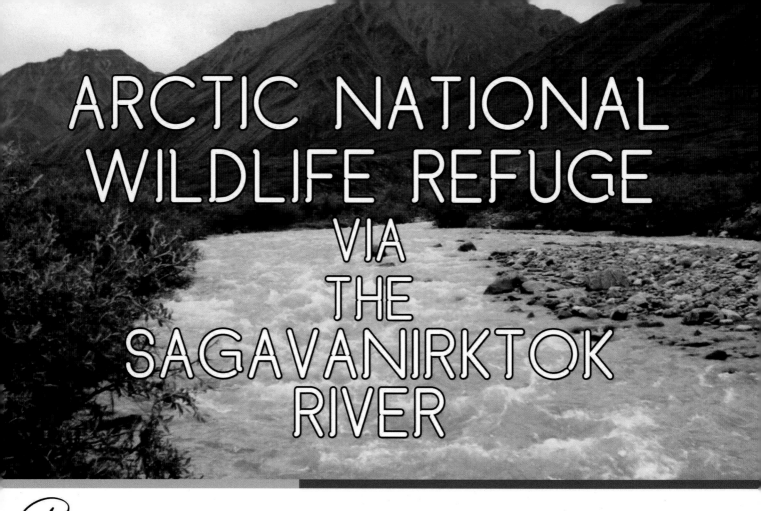

ARCTIC NATIONAL WILDLIFE REFUGE
VIA THE SAGAVANIRKTOK RIVER

By the 1980s I had been to Alaska more than fifty times and had seen most of the natural wonders of that north American continent state. One of the last remaining parts of Alaska I had not visited was the northeast area comprising the Arctic National Wildlife Refuge (ANWR). The ANWR consists of approximately 20 million acres in the Alaskan North Slope region. It is the largest national wildlife refuge in the country, slightly larger than the Yukon Delta National Wildlife Refuge. The National Wildlife Refuge System was founded by President Theodore Roosevelt in 1903 to protect areas of wildlife and wetlands in the United States.

ANWR has been surrounded in controversy since its creation due to the discovery of oil in the area and has been a political hot potato since 1977 between those who support drilling and the recovery of resources in the area and those who want to preserve the wildlife and land for future generations.

The creation of ANWR really began in 1929 when Bob Marshall, a twenty-eight year old forester, visited the upper Koyukuk River and the central Brooks Range in what was then a most unknown section of Alaska. Marshall was famous for his book Alaska Village about the small village of Wiseman which I visited in the winter by dogsled which is described in another chapter.

Marshall became quite an advocate for the protection of the north slope of Alaska because of its unique aesthetic qualities. In 1930 Marshall published an essay in the *Scientific Monthly* in defense of preserving the area: "There is just one hope of repulsing the tyrannical ambition of civilization to conquer every niche on the whole earth. That hope is the organization of spirited people who will fight for the freedom of wilderness." Marshall's efforts and his writings were a much-quoted call to action in the late twentieth century. Marshall saw the preservation of the arctic lands as "not another chance to keep chasing America's so-called destiny but a chance to finally stop chasing it." Even for Americans who had never traveled there he "thought they would benefit knowing that it still existed in the condition it always had ... In Alaska alone," Marshall wrote, "can the emotional values of the frontier be preserved?"

In 1954 the National Park Service recommended that the untouched area of the north eastern region of Alaska be preserved for research and protection of nature. The region first became a federal protected area in 1960 by the secretary of the interior under President Dwight D. Eisenhower. In 1980 congress passed the Alaskan National Interest Lands Conservation Act which was signed into law by Jimmy Carter on December 2, 1980 creating ANWR.

Currently there are no roads within or leading into the refuge. The refuge supports an amazing diversity of animal and plant life within six different eco zones that span its north to south range. The refuge is home to 37 species of land animals, 8 marine mammals including the polar bear, 42 fish species, and more than 200 migratory birds that fly there from the world over to raise their young. The only real access into the refuge is by airplane. Some of the creatures who inhabit the refuge are moose, polar bears, foxes, beavers, lynxes, martens, red foxes, river otters, porcupines, muskrats, bears, wolverines, minks and wolves. Along the north coast of the refuge are the barrier islands, coastal lagoons, salt marshes and river deltas of the arctic coastal tundra which provide habitat for thousands of migratory water birds including sea ducks, geese, swans and shorebirds. Fish such as dolly varden, grayling and arctic char are found in the inland streams. The arctic coastal plane stretches south from the coast to the foothills of the Brooks Range. The area consists of rolling hills, small lakes and north-flowing braided rivers dominated by tundra vegetation consisting of low shrubs, sedges and mosses. Caribou travel to the coastal plane during June and July to give birth and raise their young. Migratory birds and insects flourish there during the brief arctic summer. Tens of thousands of snow geese stop here during September to feed before migrating south, and the prehistoric muskox live in the refuge year-round. South of the coastal plane the mountains of the eastern Brooks Range rise to over 9,000 feet. The streams are all north-flowing and empty into the Arctic Ocean. During the summer peregrine falcons and eagles build their nests on cliffs. Harlequin ducks and red-breasted mergansers are seen on cliffs and on the river. Dall sheep, musk ox and wolf packs are active all year round. Grizzly bears and arctic ground squirrels are seen during the summer months but hibernate in the winter. The coastal plane encompasses much of the porcupine caribou herd caving grounds. Migratory caribou herds are named after their birthing grounds, in this case the Porcupine River which runs through a large part of the range of the porcupine herd. Polar Bears migrate along the 800 mile north Alaskan and Canadian coast to mate and give birth to their cubs.

I had always wanted to visit ANWR and in 1995 Margaret, my wife, and Lisa, my daughter, and I planned a kayak trip to see the Arctic National Wildlife Refuge. As I learned through much experience in Alaska the best way to see the country is to kayak, canoe or raft its rivers. My research led me to believe that the Sagavanirktok River, which flows north out of the Brooks Range and discharges into the Beaufort Sea near Prudhoe Bay and crosses the refuge, was the way to go.

Flying into the Sagavanirktok River

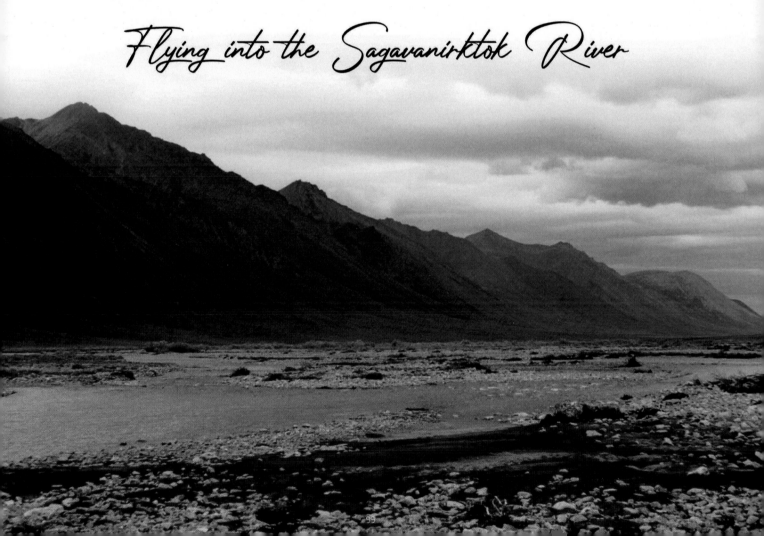

We made arrangements again with the Sourdough Outfitters in Bettles to outfit our trip. Again we flew from Bakersfield to Seattle and then to Fairbanks where we stopped for the night. We arrived in Bettles on July 16, 1995 and met up with our friends David Ketcher and his wife Tammy and son Brandon who still ran the Trading Post. We enjoyed a pleasant dinner and evening with our Alaskan friends and caught up on all the local gossip about ANWR, oil development, politics and the future of Alaska.

The next morning, after a hearty breakfast, we assembled in the shed at the trading post to organize our gear: tents, boats, food, clothing, fishing equipment, fuel for the week-long kayak trip down the Sagavanirktok River. We weren't going to take the river all the way to the Arctic Ocean since there was no pick-up there. The plan was to be picked up on the Dalton Highway that ran from Fairbanks to Prudhoe Bay and came close to the Sagavanirktok River near its discharge into the Prudhoe Bay. Pick-up by the Dalton Highway would result in a minimum of portaging our gear from the river to the pick-up vehicle.

The Dalton Highway was originally built to support the construction of the Trans-Alaska Pipeline in the mid 1970s. From Fairbanks that road was gravel for 416 miles to Anaktuvuk Pass.

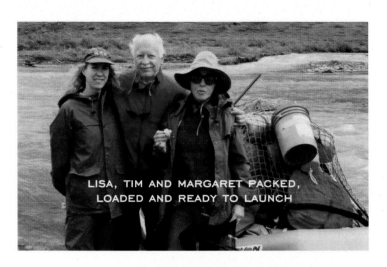

LISA, TIM AND MARGARET PACKED, LOADED AND READY TO LAUNCH

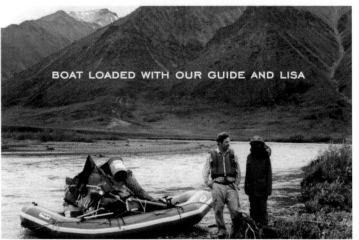

BOAT LOADED WITH OUR GUIDE AND LISA

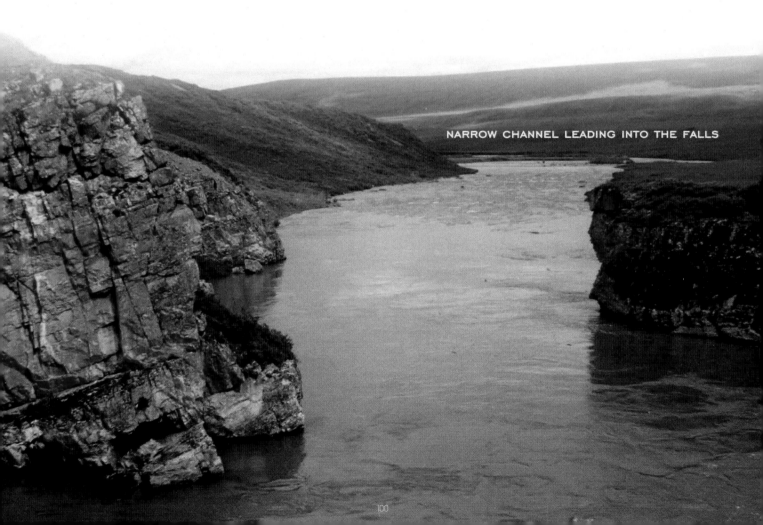

NARROW CHANNEL LEADING INTO THE FALLS

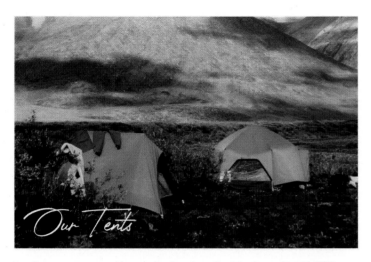

Our Tents

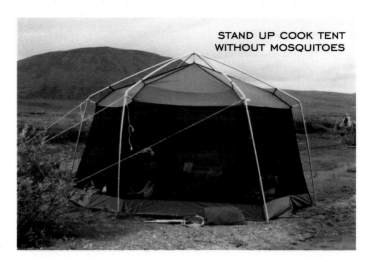

STAND UP COOK TENT
WITHOUT MOSQUITOES

It does not pass through the Arctic National Wildlife Refuge but runs close enough to the Sagavanirtok River that one can do a short portage from the river to the road and be picked up. The Dalton Highway was named after James William Dalton, an engineer who was involved in early oil exploration on the north slope. It is sometimes referred to as the Haul Road because it was used to haul supplies to build the Alaska pipeline. Neither one would exist without the other. Conservationists have resisted attempts by the federal and Alaska governments to pave the road since it would bring more people to the wilderness areas of Alaska. The road was finished in 1974. Actually hundreds of trucks use it daily to bring supplies and heavy equipment to Alaska's oil and gas fields. Although much of it still remains gravel-surfaced the sections that are paved tend to be riddled with potholes that are difficult to avoid. The highway has a formidable reputation for smashing windshields and shredding tires which is why travelers are encouraged to bring not one but two spares with them on the road. Gas stations and repairs are extremely limited, and cell phone coverage is almost nonexistent. Until the early 1980s most of the road was reserved for truckers, and public traffic was permitted only as far as Post 56 where the Dalton Highway crosses the Yukon River.

On the morning we were scheduled to leave Bettles we were packing up our gear in the Sourdough shed where we met the guide that was going to be with us for the following week. This apparently was our guide's first trip down the Sagavanirktok River although he had experience on other rivers in the Brooks Range. While we were packing our gear another guide came in and started up a friendly conversation. He asked me where we were going, and I told him that we were going to kayak the Sagavanirktok River. He looked somewhat astonished and asked our guide what kind of kayaks you are going to use. Our guide said that we were going to take canoes not kayaks. The visiting friendly guide said, "You can't take canoes or kayaks down the Sagavanirktok River." Our guide looked somewhat astonished and said, "Why not?" The response was,

"Because there are some serious falls about halfway down the river that I don't think you can get through with canoes or kayaks."

After a short discussion there was a considerable amount of exchange with our guide and some other guides that were present. A decision was quickly made that we were not going to take kayaks or canoes but rather rubber rafts down the river. I had taken many other trips on Alaska rivers with rubber rafts which are usually large enough for two people and some gear depending on how they are loaded. In retrospect we were fortunate to have this conversation with the visiting guide because of what we encountered and furthermore fortunate to have Sourdough Outfitters be able to change boats without any delay.

After the change in boating we packed up everything on the dock at the Koyukuk River, boarded a Dehaviland Beaver bush plane equipped with pontoons and took off from Bettles at about 4:00 p.m. destined for ANWR.

The flight into the Sagavanirktok River was approximately an hour and a half and we again flew over the magnificent vistas of the Brooks Range, one of the most scenic areas of Alaska. We landed on a small lake taxiing to the south end where the water was shallow enough that we could walk off the pontoons of the float plane in our hip boots.

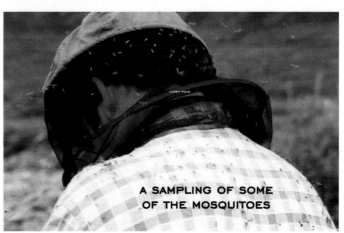

A SAMPLING OF SOME
OF THE MOSQUITOES

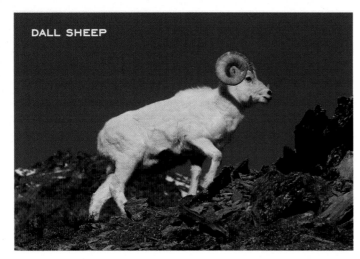
DALL SHEEP

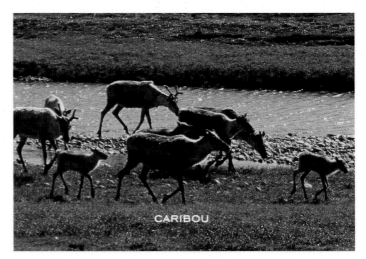
CARIBOU

We were greeted by the ubiquitous hoards of mosquitoes that one can expect in Alaska particularly in ANWR and quickly donned our mosquito netting.

Camp was set up on the south shore of the lake, a short distance from the Sagavanirktok River. We had a cooking tent that allowed one to stand erect and had collapsible chairs for each of us so that we could sit down in the tent after getting set up and ridding the tent of mosquitoes.

After depositing us and our equipment the pilot returned to the plane, took off and we were left again alone in the arctic wilderness in the middle of the Arctic National Wildlife Refuge - far removed from the trappings of civilization.

That evening we watched a moose swim across the lake that we were camped on. We had some rain squalls and a few lightening strikes. We were treated with a steak dinner and a bottle of wine, a relaxing repast after a hectic day. A magnificent double rainbow appeared in the sky and stayed in place for approximately a half hour. I felt it was a good omen. Since it was July in the arctic it didn't get dark with the sun only dimming about 2:00 or 3:00 in the morning. The immenseness of the north slope became apparent.

That night we had a very restful sleep in the cool balmy air free from the mosquitoes in our tents. The next morning we were up at 7:30 am and Lisa and I fished the lake. I caught one nice 16 inch arctic char which we fileted and fried for a delicious breakfast with scrambled eggs.

We spent the morning packing all of our gear into the rubber rafts that we had inflated. Our guide then pulled the rafts by rope down a surging creek to the Sagavanirktok where we made sure everything was securely fastened down, got positioned and took off into the river.

The Sagavanirktok name comes from the Eskimo or Inupiaq language meaning "strong current". As it turned out this was an appropriate name for the river. In the first part of the trip the water was running high, wild and wide from the rain the night before, and we had a bumpy and splashy ride down braided, shallow rapids in the clear, fast water. We moved along quite rapidly in the surging stream that was high from the thirty to forty minute downpour the evening before. We entered a long lush, green valley with no trees and only willows along the banks, the highest being no more than ten feet. The treeless region was tundra-covered permafrost.

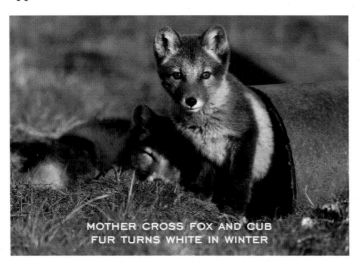
MOTHER CROSS FOX AND CUB
FUR TURNS WHITE IN WINTER

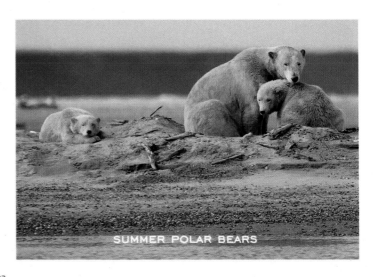
SUMMER POLAR BEARS

We were treated with the sight of three wolves running along the bank, following us down the river barking and howling. Their barking and howling caused other wolves in the vicinity to join in. Our guide figured out we must have disturbed a den because there were a number of wolves, all very large and healthy looking creatures, the epitome of Alaska wilderness.

We also passed a red fox running along the cut bank above us for many yards starring at us curiously wondering what in the world we were doing in his home.

The scenery was immense, wide open and magnificent, the land expanse enormous. We stopped for a leisurely lunch on a sand bar and enjoyed the scenery with some hot cups of soup. Cruising down the river with the current moving us along now at a slower float since the river had calmed somewhat gave us ample time to absorb the beauty, the enormity and the remoteness of the Alaskan wildlife refuge. We were moving through country scarcely visited by humans, unchanged, and in the condition it has always been.

That night we camped on a sandy rocky beach with a nice wind that kept the mosquitoes at bay. We had good tenting equipment because it rained practically all night, at times very heavily, and we were cozy and warm in our tents. We stayed dry and slept well in our warm sleeping bags on air mattresses. The next morning when we got up it looked like the river had come up at least a foot or more. It was not real cold, but it was cool with broken clouds blowing through the area. Since it was still raining we stayed in our sleeping bags and slept in, again warm and not bothered by mosquitoes.

On July 17th we were treated to the sight of Alaskan Muskox, a prehistoric beast that lives in the Arctic National Wildlife Refuge all year around. The muskox is a stocky long-haired animal with a shoulder hump and a short tail. Eskimos call the animal Itomingmak, meaning "the animal with skin like a beard" in reference to the long guard hair that hangs nearly to the ground. Both male and female muskox have horns, but the horns of the bulls are larger and hairier than those of the cows. The horns of bulls develop large bosses which nearly span their entire forehead. The mature bulls are about 5 feet high and weight 600 to 800 pounds. Cows are smaller averaging 4 feet and weighing 400 to 500 pounds. At the close of the last ice age muskoxen were found across northern Europe, Asia, Greenland and North America including Alaska. By the mid 1800s they had disappeared from Europe and Asia and by the 1920s had disappeared from Alaska probably because of over-hunting. In 1930 muskoxen were captured in Greenland and brought back to Alaska to the Arctic National Wildlife Refuge

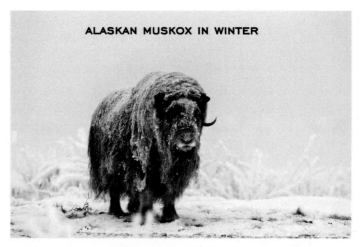

ALASKAN MUSKOX IN WINTER

where they have prospered. Battles between bull muskoxen during the rut are spectacular and violent contests. After a period of aggressive display the bulls charge at top speed from distances of 50 yards or more and collide squarely on the horn bosses. The sound can be heard from a mile away on a calm day. After a clash the bulls back away from each other swinging their heads from side to side and repeat the sequence until one bull turns and runs. The battle may include 20 clashes. Bull muskoxen have heavily armored skulls to protect them from the shock of the impact. 4 inches of horn and 3 inches of bone lie directly over the brain in the area of contact. It is astonishing how these animals can survive on the north slope of Alaska in the brutal winter season where the temperature can fall to 60 below 0. Winters last eight to nine months with only three short months of summer when the temperature can reach into the 90s.

By July 18th we arrived in the area where the falls we had been warned of were located. We had to unload our boats and line the boats down along the shore through big boulders with long ropes. It was slow going since the guide and I had to portage most of the equipment around the cliffs and down to the new takeout location. We lined the boats approximately a quarter of a mile down the river where we came to the falls. This was approximately a 15 foot fall. I would classify the rapid as a V.

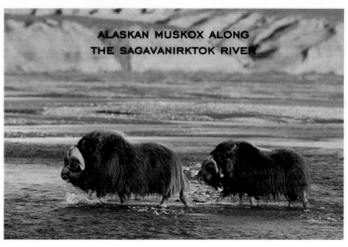

ALASKAN MUSKOX ALONG
THE SAGAVANIRKTOK RIVER

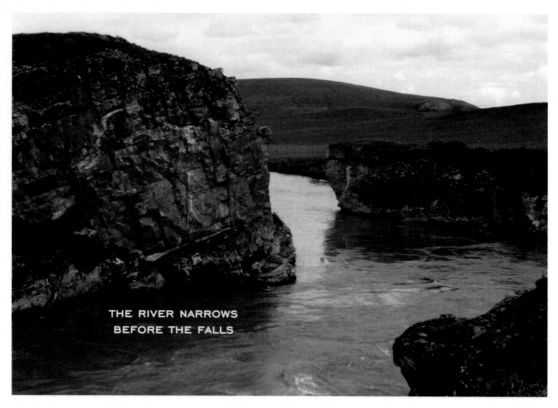

THE RIVER NARROWS
BEFORE THE FALLS

I do not think there was any way that we could have taken a kayak or canoe down through these falls. You could take rubber rafts down through there but it would be a hazardous experience and the danger of capsizing would be significant. Had we gone down the river in canoes and not been aware of the falls there is no doubt that we would have capsized and lost a lot of our gear. At the falls the river flowed into a narrow gorge, 20 to 30 feet across, forcing all water over a rock ledge with a 10 to 15 foot drop.

At the bottom of the drop was a whirling whirlpool backwash with the current smashing into the rocks on the right bank. After the falls the river went through a narrow channel with vertical cliffs some 50 feet high on each side.

Our guide Chris was a white water guide and experienced rafter and canoeist and said there was absolutely no way we could have come through there with kayaks or canoes. He would not even take an empty raft down the falls which meant we had to carry the rafts and all the gear around the falls. We had no choice but to unload the rafts completely at the small beach above the falls and portage everything around the falls. In order to do this we had to climb over a steep bank and around rocky outcroppings and scramble down a steep bank to a location where we could again load the rafts.

It was a long tedious day portaging all the baggage to the new put-in location. Chris and I had to hand-carry everything and reload all the rafts. Once we were loaded up we were underway again.

On Wednesday, July 19, 1995 we slept in again because it was raining in the morning and we were dry and cozy in our sleeping bags and we didn't want to be out on the river in the rain. After breakfast the rain had stopped and Lisa and I hiked to a lake to the west over a ridge above our camp. The hike was slow going in the sloggy tusks and tundra. The lake didn't have a name but it was a large beautiful lake.

At the shore of the lake we followed a moose and caribou trail out to a point in the lake where I tried some fishing. I tried three locations without any response. I was not sure that there were any fish in the lake although Chris said that he had caught char there in the past. The lake was fairly shallow, and it probably freezes solid in most places in the winter. Lisa and I returned to camp and Margaret and Chris were packing up. We helped them and by 2:30 we were on our way on the river again. It was late in the day and we hit a long series of rapids, some quite large, and all got somewhat soaked. We had to pull over the shore twice to bail out the rafts. It was getting cold and windy and raining off and on and everyone was wet and uncomfortable. We camped at the juncture of Accomplishment Creek and Sagavan-irktok River. I tried fishing again but the water was

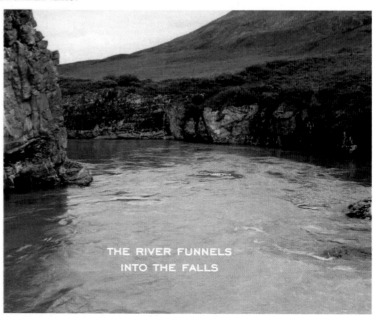

THE RIVER FUNNELS
INTO THE FALLS

too high from rain and no luck. Later in the afternoon the fog started rolling in from the Beaufort Sea bringing cold and rain. We had our camp set up and got in our tents because it rained steadily all night - from 11:00 p.m. to 9:00 a.m.

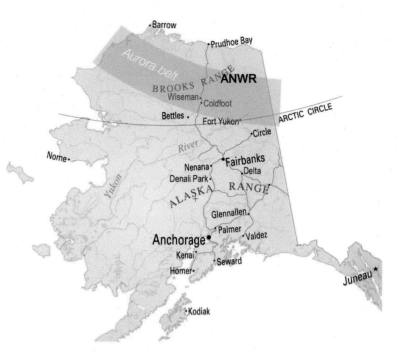

On Thursday, July 20, 1995 the rain had stopped. The bugs were tolerable. It was still foggy and overcast. This was going to be the last day before takeout and we had approximately six miles to the takeout location near the Dalton Highway or the Haul Road. Chris warned us that there would be white water on the way and we would probably get wet again. Accomplishment Creek was running at high flood stage and pushing the Sagavanirktok River against its west bank. It had rained all night and was still raining sporadically in the morning as we packed up our wet camp to leave.

By the time we finished packing it was 2:00 p.m. and we started down the swollen Sagavanirktok River and ran into some class III "brown water." It was cold and windy and in the rain and wind the mosquitoes swarmed around us unabated. It was slow going for the last six miles to the takeout point which was called Maintenance Camp on the Haul Road.

In the last run of rapids before Maintenance Camp I got thoroughly soaked. I took a big wave in the face and it splashed down my neck to soak me and my clothes down to my stomach and to my underwear. The rapids contained some rather large rocks that Chris called "raft eaters." Chris, however, expertly maneuvered around the rocks.

By 3:00 p.m. we had reached the maintenance camp on the Haul Road. We pulled the rafts out of the river and set up our cook tent for shelter to get out of the rain and avoid the ubiquitous mosquitoes. We prepared some hot soup and snacks. After changing into warm clothes our attitudes were greatly improved. At Maintenance Camp we were to be picked up by a driver who was going to take us back down the Dalton Highway to Coldfoot, the nearest settlement.

One driver, Norman, a true Alaskan character, arrived at 3:30 p.m., a typical Alaska time miscalculation. Norman told us that he formerly resided in Oklahoma when God told him to move to Wiseman, Alaska. He was a minister and in Wiseman he and his wife lived in a 16'x16' cabin that served as their home, a church, school and community meeting place. Being new to Alaska Margaret asked him: "What is the most unusual thing you have seen since coming to Alaska?" he replied: "I have never married a couple where the groom was wearing wading boots." With Norman we drove 150 miles back to Coldfoot being entertained the whole way by Norman's storytelling about Alaska life and his ministry. He obviously had not had much social contact in the last few months and regaled us with his Alaska tales.

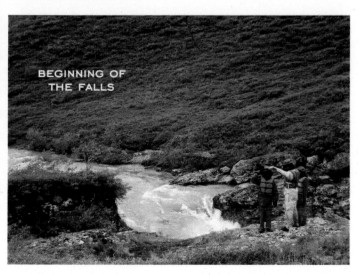

BEGINNING OF THE FALLS

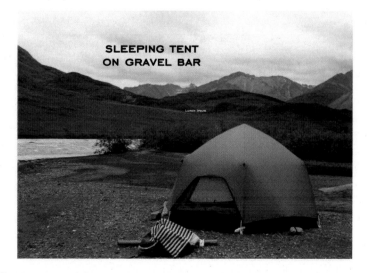

SLEEPING TENT ON GRAVEL BAR

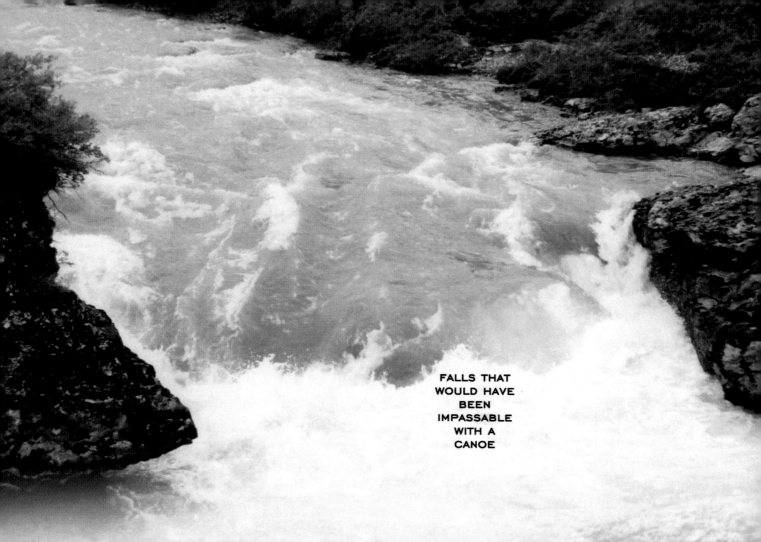

FALLS THAT
WOULD HAVE
BEEN
IMPASSABLE
WITH A
CANOE

Coldfoot is on the Dalton Highway and is known as the northernmost truck stop in the world and the last place with gas and services before the 240 mile stretch to Dead Horse or Prudhoe Bay where the Haul Road comes to an end on the Arctic coast. Coldfoot's origins relate back to the 1890s when prospectors came there in search of gold. The famous story is that they got this far and realized it was going to be really cold and turned around and left. "They got cold feet. Thus the place became Coldfoot Camp."

After gold was discovered in nearby Wiseman, Coldfoot was largely abandoned by the 1920s.

In the 1970s the town gained new life as a camp for workers building the trans-Alaska pipeline. By the 1980s it became a regular stop for truckers on the Daltan Highway thanks in the large part to the efforts of Iditarod champion Dick Mackey. Dick Mackey was the father of Bill Mackey, my dogsled guide through the gates of the Arctic National Park. I took three long distance dogsled trips with Bill Mackey which I describe in another chapter.

When Dick Mackey originally came to Coldfoot all he had was a bus that he heated with a stove. He served burgers and coffees out of the back of his bus and the truckers loved it. The truckers loved it so much that Mackey decided to build a permanent truck stop using surplus materials from the trucks bound for the north slope.

In the times that I have been there Coldfoot boasts a restaurant, a U.S. post office and some trailers put together as an inn. There is an airstrip there that can be used in the summer and in the winter for a plane equipped with skis.

When Norman left us at Coldfoot we rented a room at the Coldfoot Inn at $125.00 per night. We were able to take showers and eat at the restaurant. The next morning we were up at 6:30, had a hearty breakfast at the Coldfoot Truck Stop, were ferried by truck over to the airport strip to wait for the commuter plane from Fairbanks that would arrive between 10:00 and 12:00. The plane came and we loaded and were on our way back to Fairbanks and home.

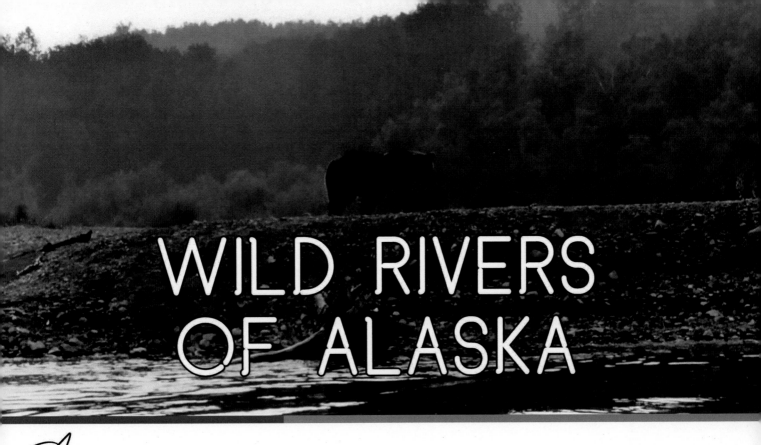

WILD RIVERS OF ALASKA

After my trips down the Noatak and the Stikine River it became apparent to me that one of the best ways to experience the untapped wilderness of Alaska was to float, kayak or canoe some of its wild rivers. Over the next 20 or more years I had the opportunity to experience many of them.

∽ LAKE CREEK YETNA RIVER ∽

One of the most pleasant Alaska wild river trips was one to Lake Creek in south central Alaska in 1982. This was a trip I took with cousin Clyde Barbeau, Dewy Seales, Don Galey, and Jack Moffett The trip started in Anchorage where we took a float plane from Hood Lake, the central float plane lake in Anchorage, flew across the Cook Inlet and basically followed the Yetna River and then turned north heading toward the Chelatna Lake which is the head waters of the Lake Creek River. It is called Lake Creek but it is actually a pretty good size river. It is famous for its great salmon runs as well as having a variety of fish. It has both a king and silver salmon run as well as good sized rainbow trout and dolly varden. King salmon use Lake Creek and Chelatna as a spawning site and return in large numbers each year. Lake Creek is a clear swift stream with class III and IV rapids with many technical boulders to get around. For the large boulders in the stream you need to have some solid rafting and paddling skills to circumvent them without capsizing.

We learned this the first day when the raft with Clyde Barbeau and Don Galey was sucked down by a big boulder in the stream and overturned causing us to spend several hours collecting the gear that had spilled out of their raft and was swept down the river by the current.

The flight into Lake Creek was a usual Alaska, "wow" with big views of Mt. Denali and Foraker, two of the most magnificent peaks in the Alaska range. Our pilot took a few minutes to fly up toward Denali to get some fantastic views of these enormous mountains. After circling around and reveling in the scenery we headed our float plane back towards Chelatna Lake, landed smoothly and taxied to the Chelatna Lodge on the south end of the lake.

The first evening at the lodge we were treated by the visit of a mother moose and two newborn calves feeding on the swampy vegetation on the banks of the lake. We were able to carefully walk slowly up to where the mother and the two youngsters were eating without spooking them to get some great pictures. We were warned not to get too close because a mother moose can be very protective of their offspring and can charge an intruder and do great damage. That night we had a typical Alaskan feast with plenty of good Napa Valley wine that we brought with us.

The next morning we loaded all of our equipment onto three rubber rafts each to carry two men plus their gear. There were six of us all together including our guide. We had to line the rafts down the shallow creek exiting Chelatna Lake into Lake Creek. As the water got higher we were able to paddle down the outlet and exit into Lake Creek which was flowing swiftly. As indicated Barbeau and Galey capsized their raft on the first morning strewing their equipment all over the river which took some time to clean up.

We took this trip three years in a row because we enjoyed it so much. The fishing was great for trout salmon and dolly varden. We ate a lot of the fish that we would catch both for breakfast and dinner. The first year we went the king and silver salmon had not started running on their egg laying frenzy up the creek but there were a few early fish we were able to hook. Each trip that we took on Lake Creek was about five days in length. The guide had selected pre-determined places for our night time camps, most had canvas tents already erected and stretched out over poles held in place with ties. Since it rained usually everyday the tents were high enough that one could stand erect, and they also gave you a place to sleep at night that was dry. The entire course of the trip down Lake Creek was only about seventy miles, and we camped approximately four times and enjoyed the leisure of the camp with the beautiful views of Mt. Denali and Mt. Foraker and the Kahiltna glacier in the north. At each camp we usually had an outdoor fire and when it was not raining could sit around the fire in lounge chairs enjoying our wine after a hearty meal. On each trip we were the only people that were on the river, so it was like our own and private stream.

The first camp after leaving Chelatna Lake was at Sunflower Creek, a known good fishing spot, where we had really excellent fishing and by this time catching and releasing most of the trout since we had plenty to eat.

Our third camp was at Camp Creek about fifteen miles into the trip, and our fourth camp at Home Creek at twenty miles into the trip. At about twelve miles down Lake Creek we hit our first set of significant rapids. They were really not that bad, and we followed each other down through the rapids with some splashing and wetness but with nothing serious. Fortunately, no one capsized.

On our last trip down Lake Creek two years later in 1986 we did run into some serious problems because of a significant downpour that caused the river to swell considerably. It rained quite hard for two days and the river got so high and swift that we decided we better spend the night at a camp on a high bank and wait for the river to mellow out before heading down to the Yetna River. At our last camp on the banks at Home Creek the river had actually risen about five feet and was threatening to flood our tents and sleeping bags.

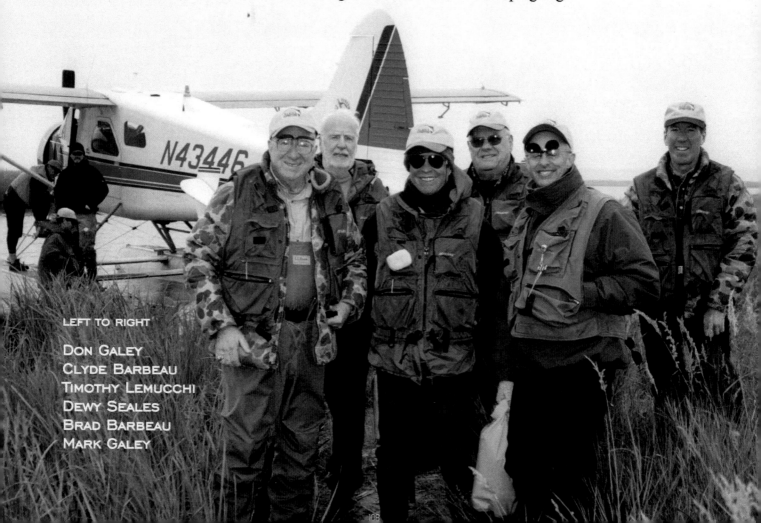

LEFT TO RIGHT

DON GALEY
CLYDE BARBEAU
TIMOTHY LEMUCCHI
DEWY SEALES
BRAD BARBEAU
MARK GALEY

That's when we decided we had better find a place to camp high enough above the river to keep dry and wait for it to retreat before going down to the Yetna River and our takeout location.

Our guide knew where there was an old miner's cabin, and we pulled into a small stream outlet where we could securely anchor our boats to the trees. We had to carry all of our equipment - sleeping bags, cooking equipment and food - up to the cabin. Even though this was an abandoned somewhat dilapidated rustic old cabin we were able to prepare a good hot meal on a stove that was still in the cabin and dry off. While we transported our goods to the cabin and prepared our meal it continued to rain heavily. Fortunately we retrieved our beer and wine from the cooler in the boats and the evening passed quite pleasantly.

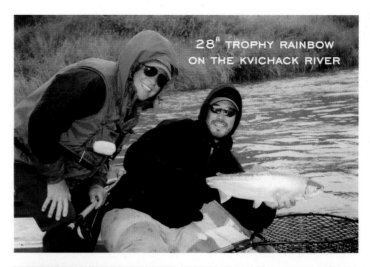

28" TROPHY RAINBOW ON THE KVICHACK RIVER

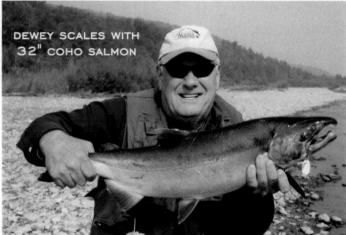

DEWEY SCALES WITH 32" COHO SALMON

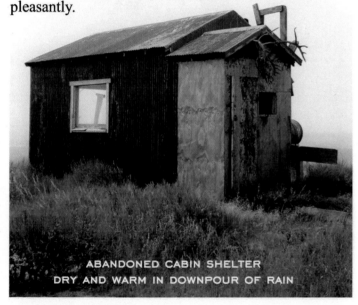

ABANDONED CABIN SHELTER
DRY AND WARM IN DOWNPOUR OF RAIN

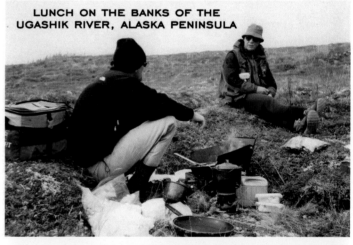

LUNCH ON THE BANKS OF THE UGASHIK RIVER, ALASKA PENINSULA

At night the rain did calm down somewhat and the river began to recede slowly the next morning. Although, it was still running quite high and looked somewhat dangerous for a small raft.

The next day, our fifth day out, we rafted down to the Yetna River which is a fairly large river at least three times the size of Lake Creek. The Yetna runs into the Susitna River which is one of Alaska's major rivers and basically drains the high mountains of the Alaska range. Our plan was to raft down the Yetna to a previously agreed on takeout point at a guide's cabin about a half day of rafting from where Lake Creek merged into the Yetna. We reached the guide's cabin without any problems although the Yetna was also running high and swift. The guide had a boat dock on the river and we were able to unload all of our equipment onto the deck. We pulled our boats up, deflated them and flattened them out. The boats were to be picked up by guides on another trip. Later on that day we were picked up by a prearranged float plane and flown back to Anchorage. Our trip on Lake Creek was approximately 70 miles.

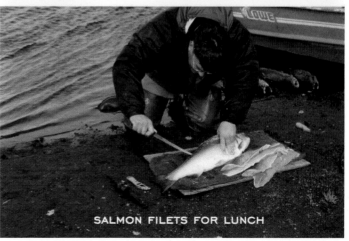

SALMON FILETS FOR LUNCH

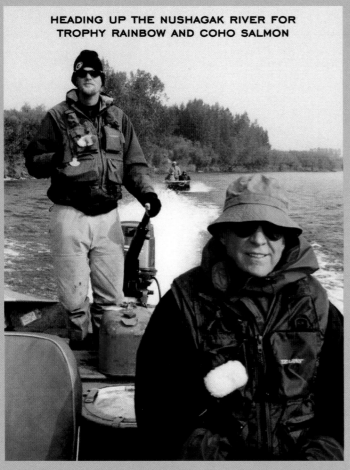

HEADING UP THE NUSHAGAK RIVER FOR TROPHY RAINBOW AND COHO SALMON

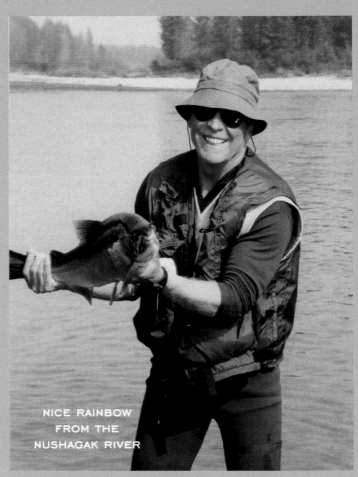

NICE RAINBOW FROM THE NUSHAGAK RIVER

The Fishing was Quite Good

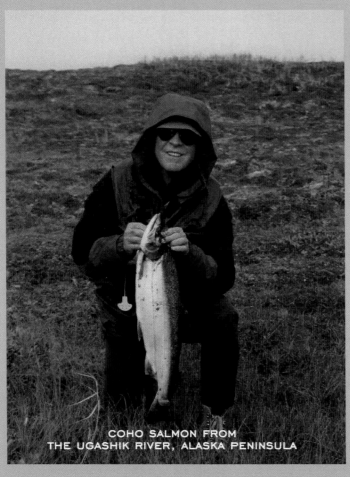

COHO SALMON FROM THE UGASHIK RIVER, ALASKA PENINSULA

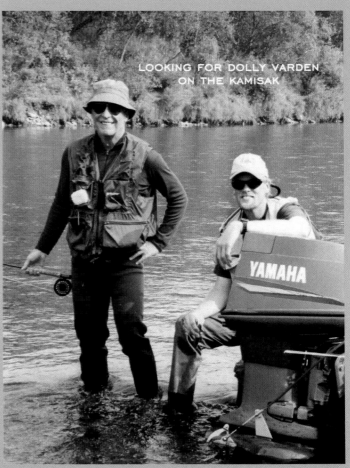

LOOKING FOR DOLLY VARDEN ON THE KAMISAK

ᗰ MULCHATNA RIVER ᗰ

Our next wild river trip was on the big Mulchatna River. On that trip was Don Galey, Jack Moffat and myself. Barbeau was unable to attend that year. We had heard about a guide who had a remote cabin on the western flank of the Alaska Range from my good friend Bill Juvonen. Through our research we learned that the Mulchatna River passed through some of the most untouched wilderness in Alaska so we decided to give it a try. Again we started our trip from Anchorage and were were picked up at Hood Lake, the sea plane lake in Anchorage that is used by most guides to fly into the wilderness. We took off from Hood Lake and flew across the Knik Inlett toward the Alaska Range. The Knick arm is a waterway and one of the two branches of the Cook Inlett, the other being Turnagin arm. The Port of Anchorage is located on the Knik arm. As we flew across the Knik arm we passed over the Susitna River, the largest stream emptying into the inlett and is in the area where we fished at Lake Creek. After crossing the Knik Inlett we headed toward the Alaska Range and the infamous Merrill Pass which is the lowest small airline pass in the Alaska Range. Because of sudden and unpredictable turbulence and up-drafts the pass has a reputation for taking the lives of unskilled pilots and you can see when you are flying through the pass the wreckage of may float planes on the sides of the mountains. That year as we crossed the pass you could see an upside down float plane in a small lake toward the head of the pass. Passing through Merrill Pass not too many feet above the Alaska range we headed to the guide's cabin at a small lake on the west side of the range, landing the float plane on the lake without any problem and taxing across the lake to the guide's cabin. He had built a rustic cabin on the shore of the lake with a couple of small chalets that we used for bedrooms. Each of the bedrooms had the beds covered with animal furs - fox, bear and lynx. We were treated the first night to a freshly killed moose meat dinner which was extraordinarily good. The next day we took off again in the float plane and headed toward the Mulchatna River landing in the river channel at a predetermined spot where the guide had stationed two rubber rafts for our trip. We unloaded the plane and got our rafts loaded with all of our equipment. Our guide was to stay with us through the five day trip and the pilot to would pick us up at a predetermined spot down the river.

The Mulchatna River is one of Alaska's wild and scenic rivers specifically noted for the good fishing, all types of salmon, trout, grayling and arctic char. Its headwaters are at the Turquoise Lake along the western edge of the Neocola Mountains of the Alaska range and the river lies within the boundaries of Lake Clark National Park and Preserve. The river is seasonally high and low depending on the rainfall and travels through a swift rocky gorge with some class III rapids to negotiate. The length of the river is about 230 miles but our trip was going to be about 60 miles and take five days in our rafts. We were initially scheduled to end the trip at a place called Dummy Creek where a float plane could land. Where we landed is heavily forested in spruce and birch.

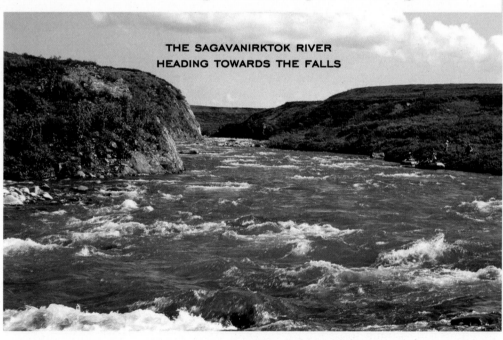

THE SAGAVANIRKTOK RIVER
HEADING TOWARDS THE FALLS

Our trip was five days camping each night on the banks of the river. The fishing was quite good and I caught a 25 inch rainbow trout which at the time was the largest rainbow I had landed which was quite a thrill.

At the conclusion of our float we were picked up again by our pilot guide in his float plane and had a rather harrowing experience returning to his cabin. We flew up over Lake Clark where it was raining quite heavily and as we started up into the canyons above Lake Clark to wind our way to the cabin the ceiling kept descending. All of us, even the pilot, were concerned about becoming trapped in one of the canyons in a low ceiling. Eventually the pilot did find his way through the descending clouds and made his way back to the lake and the cabin where we had a warm shower and another hearty Alaska dinner. Out of the presence of the pilot we all discussed the terrifying plane flight back to the cabin and drank a salute to our survival.

≈ CHILIKADROTNA RIVER ≈

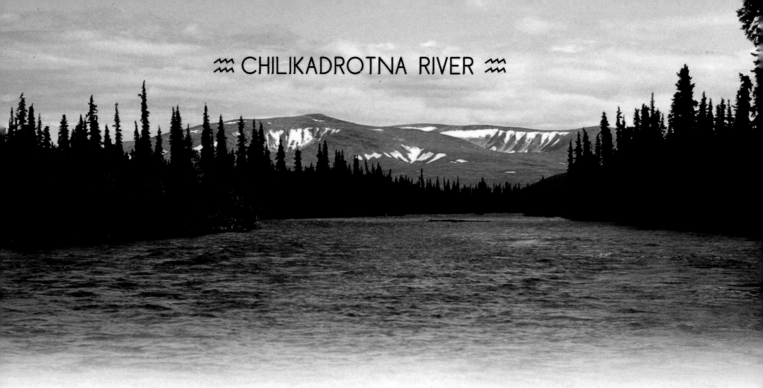

Even before the trip down the Mulchatna River we had heard considerable good information about the float of the Chilikadrotna River which is another one of Alaska's wild and scenic rivers. The Chilikadrontna River originates in the Chigmit Mountains which is a subrange of the Alaska aleutian range. The river begins at Twin Lakes and flows west through the foothills approximately 10 miles to the border of the Lake Clark National Park and Preserve and then continues an additional 35 miles before it joins the Mulchatna River. We had passed the outlet of the Chilikadrotna River into the Mulchatna River on our previous trip and thought that this would also be a good river to experience the Alaska wilderness. The very next year we signed up for Chilikadrotna trip and hired a guide who was a dentist in Anchorage. The dentist had a Twin Otter made by the de Havilland Company, the same company that makes the beaver but with two engines. It is also a float plane. Again we were picked up in Anchorage at Hood Lake by our guide and flown into the Stony River on the west side of the Alaska range where we spent the first night at the guide's cabin on the Stony River. The cabin was a beautiful place which the guide had built himself. It consisted of a large chalet with a kitchen and dining room and outside the main chalet were smaller cabins that were used as bedrooms with baths and showers. We spent a very pleasant late afternoon and evening at the Stoney River with our guide.

On this trip were my cousin Clyde Barbeau, Dewey Seals, Don Galey and myself. We planned to float the Chilikadrotna in rubber rafts and had a guide from Bakersfield that was going to stay with us on the trip.

Our main guide who arranged the trip would just fly us into the headwaters of the Chilikadrotna, drop us off and then pick us up at the end of the trip. We took off from the Stony River landing strip - a gravel bar next to the river. The Twin Otter was capable of landing both on a field and water since it had wheels under the pontoons that could be lowered for hard-pack landing. We were flown into Twin Lakes which is at the headwaters of the Chilikadrotna. We unloaded our equipment and portaged all of our gear over to the river where we loaded up and started our trip. The river has some class II/III challenges but by this time most of us had sufficient skills to avoid the sweepers, tight turns and the boulders. The river is quite beautiful - actually much more so than the Mulchatna which does run through some tundra land and not as scenic as the Chilikadrotna.

In the first part of the trip the river flows past the high peaks of Lake Clark National Park and Preserve which were still covered with snow. The river which runs at an average of 5 miles an hour travels through birch and spruce forests. There are large sand bars and gravel bars which are frequent offering plenty of places to fish and camp. There was an abundance of firewood and each night we enjoyed an outdoor fire if it was not raining. The fishing again was excellent with some salmon, rainbow, char and grayling. There was a variety of ducks, geese, occasional moose and a grizzly bear. On most of our river trips we usually had some close encounters with the grizzlies ubiquitous.

It was a great trip.

I became very familiar with the Kvichak River because the Alaska Rainbow Lodge located on the south bank of the river. Don Galey was a personal friend of Ron and Sharon Hayes who built the Alaksa Rainbow Lodge in 1982 to take advantage of its location on the Kvichak River and its proximity to the Bristol Bay, one of the most prolific fishing areas in the world. Also famous in the area are the trophy rainbow trout at the outlet to the Iliamna Lake just a few miles above the lodge and easily accessible by boat on plane from the lodge. The Kvichak River has one of the largest salmon runs in the world and sockeye salmon swim past the lodge's front door by the millions each summer. Large rainbow trout that inhabit Iliamna Lake come out of the lake into the flat lands just before the start of the

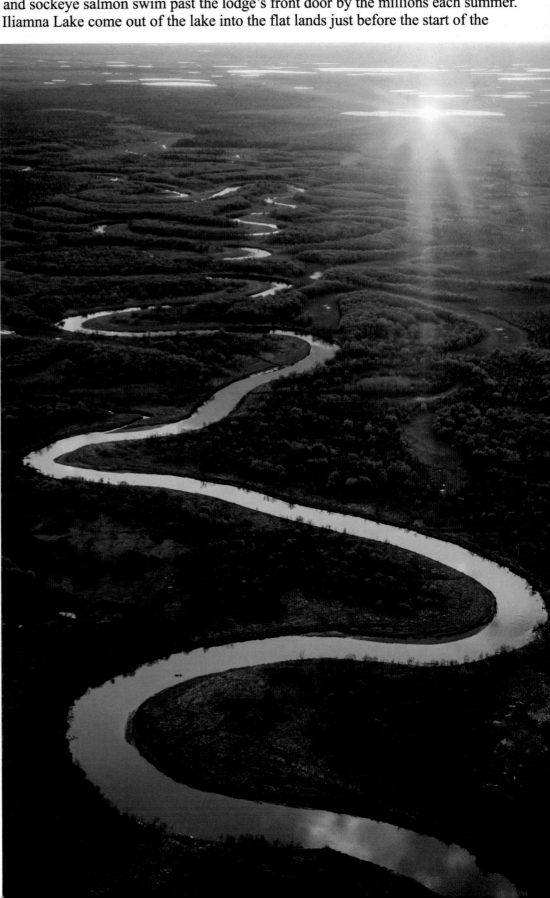

Kvichak River to consume the sockeye salmon eggs that are being laid in the riverbed by the millions. The rainbows can reach 34 inches in length and weigh up to 18 pounds. I have caught a few in the 25-30 inch range. Catching a 30 inch rainbow trout on a fly rod is quite a thrill and does take some expertise as to not lose the fish as they are so powerful they can snap your line in an instant if you don't play them correctly. All the fishing for trophy rainbow is by fly rod and is catch-and-release. The lodge only takes 16 guests and they have access to three float airplanes that can take the guests into the Alagnak River, the Kvichak River, the Nushagak River and the Naknek River within a few minutes of taking off from the Kvichak River for some of the best fishing in the world. There is an incredible king salmon run, a silver salmon run, a sockeye salmon run as well as char, dolly varden and grayling. During the 20 plus years I have stayed at the Alaska Rainbow Lodge I have had the opportunity to fish, float and boat the Kvichak, the Alagnak, Nushagnak, Naknek and other rivers that drain into the Bristol Bay - one of the top fishing areas in the world and we have always caught all the fish that we could handle.

Probably one of the most pleasant river trips that I took in the Alaska wilderness was on the Wild River with my wife, Margaret and niece Lanette Valpredo Caratan. The Wild River was a 65 mile trip through a lovely heavily forested valley beginning at the Wild Lake and ending on the Koyukuk River where it flows past the village of Bettles. This was a six day canoe trip. The Wild River is a class I river with only a few class II riffles. It is a crystal clear stream that is swift at first out of the lake and gradually slowing in current as it approaches the Koyukuk River. This trip started in Fairbanks. We took a small commuter airline into Bettles and met up with our guide at the Sourdough Trading Post for one of our last trips with Sourdough. We had booked a float plane to fly us from the dock in Bettles into the Wild Lake where we were to begin our trip. The Wild Lake is a long deep narrow lake set in a broad valley just south of the northern tree line. Sandy beaches and a white spruce forest surround the six mile lake where we landed and spend the first night on the banks of the lake.

After a warm night sleep in our sleeping bags in our tents we packed up our gear in the canoes which can hold a considerable amount of equipment and started southbound on the lake toward the outlet into the Wild River. Once we got to the outlet we started down a fairly narrow channel toward the main river. When I kayaked over 300 miles in the Noatak River I found kayaking to be very safe since the kayak being "bottom heavy" is actually difficult to tip over unless you get into rough water that rolls the kayak on its sides.

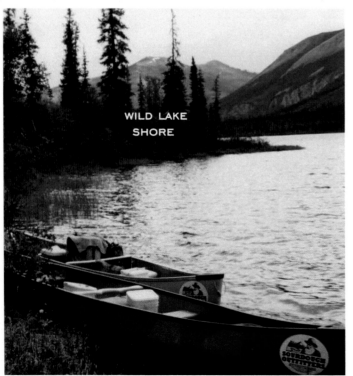

WILD LAKE
SHORE

Canoes are a different animal, at least to me. Although some people prefer the canoe because you sit up higher, in my experience a canoe is not as stable with an inexperienced partner. This was proven on the first day when both Margaret and I caused the canoe to capsize and soak my Canon camera. We were going down a narrow channel where we both unfortunately leaned to the same side to avoid a branch when we should have been leaning in the opposite direction and caused the canoe to roll over spilling all of our equipment into the stream soaking my canon camera. It took some time to collect the equipment.

I had gotten some early pictures of the trip but after the dunking of my Canon I was unable to take photographs of the remainder of the trip which of course was some of the most beautiful country. The Wild River was exceptionally beautiful and easy to maneuver on a canoe once we got the hang of the two people working together to keep the canoe in a straight line and balanced. At nights we had rain off and on but the tents that we had kept us warm and dry with warm sleeping bags. We did have a cook tent where we could stand up and close all the portals to keep the mosquitoes out so we enjoyed the time of the river. We also enjoyed eating the freshly caught trout and grayling. I had been down the Wild River on one of my dog sledding trips to the winter but then the river was iced over and topped with snow so that the surrounding country side was not easily recognizable. On the summer trip I did find some moose horns which I attached to the baggage on the canoe and brought back to Bettles and then paid the fee to have the horns shipped back to California where I hung them in our house at Mammoth Lakes.

When we returned to Fairbanks we spent another night, July 4th, before returning to California. While having dinner at the Pump House Restaurant we saw an ad that there was going to be a 10k run on July 4th beginning at midnight at the University of Alaska campus in Fairbanks. During dinner and after a couple glasses of wine we decided it would be a great idea if we all ran in the midnight run in Fairbanks. Since we finished dinner around 9:30 we had plenty of time to go back to our hotel, put on our running gear and go to the university campus where we signed up and ran in the Fairbanks Midnight Run. It was quite an experience with approximately 2,000 people in the race that wound through the campus and the town of Fairbanks and then finished at the campus where there was a midnight 4th of July celebration with a band and dancing in the still brightly shining sun. It was quite a trip.

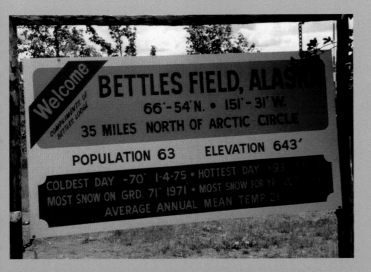

BETTLES FIELD, ALASKA
66°-54'N. • 151°-31'W.
35 MILES NORTH OF ARCTIC CIRCLE
POPULATION 63   ELEVATION 643'
COLDEST DAY -70° 1-4-75 • HOTTEST DAY +93°
MOST SNOW ON GRD. 71" 1971 • MOST SNOW FOR YR. 207"
AVERAGE ANNUAL MEAN TEMP. 21°

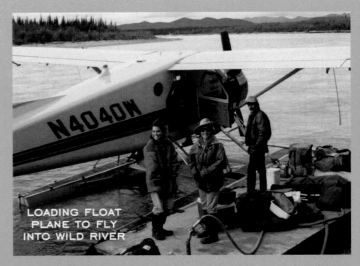

LOADING FLOAT
PLANE TO FLY
INTO WILD RIVER

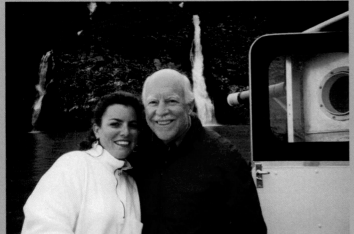

LANETTE VALPREDO CARATAN
AND TIM LEMUCCHI

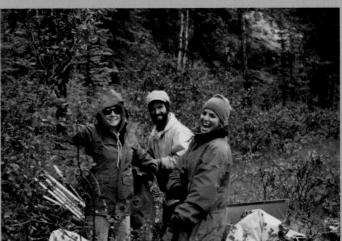

MARGARET LEMUCCHI, WILD RIVER GUIDE
AND LANETTE VALPREDO CARATAN

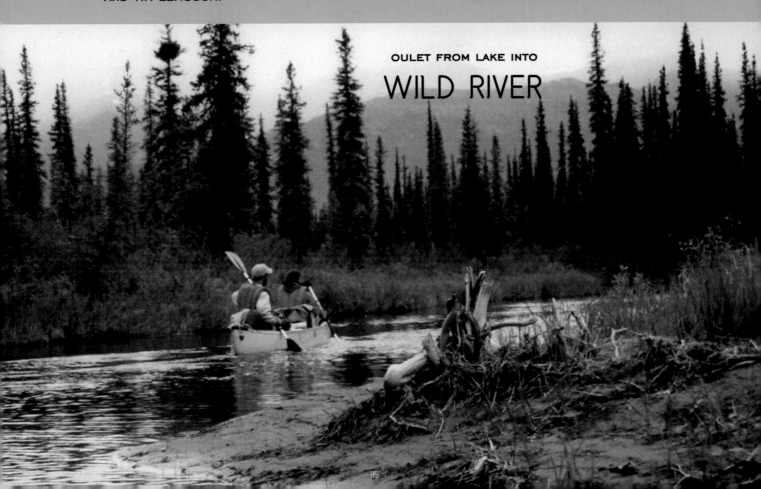

OULET FROM LAKE INTO
WILD RIVER

WILD RIVER
SIX DAY CANOE TRIP
65 MILES

PROBABLY ONE OF THE
MOST PLEASANT RIVER TRIPS
THAT I TOOK IN THE
ALASKA WILDERNESS
WAS ON THE WILD RIVER
WITH MY WIFE,
MARGARET AND NIECE
LANETTE VALPREDO CARATAN

SOURDOUGH HEADQUARTERS BETTLES, ALASKA
MARGARET, TIM & LANETTE

PARKING CANOES ON WILD RIVER

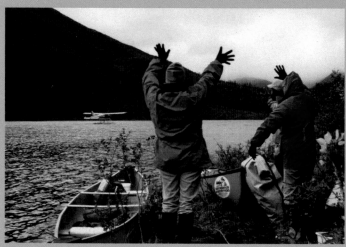

FLOAT PLANE TAKING OFF FROM WILD LAKE

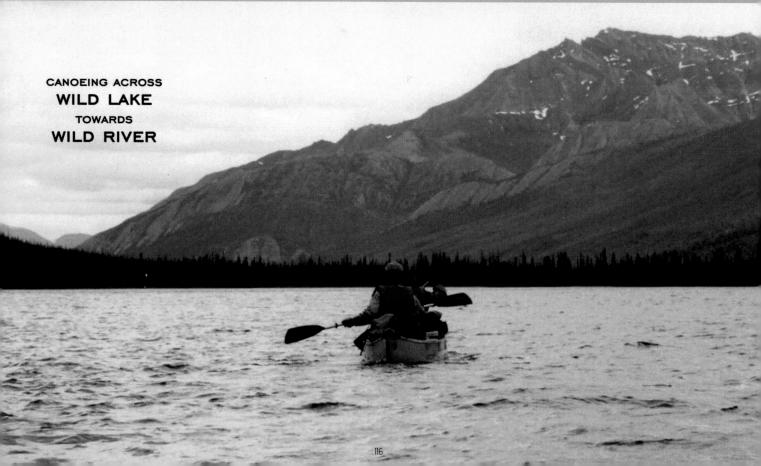

CANOEING ACROSS
WILD LAKE
TOWARDS
WILD RIVER

The Kamishak River is a long winding stream that drains from the high mountains of the Alaska Peninsula at the very top of the Katmai National Park and Preserve, a 4.3 million acre national park on the Alaska Peninsula. The Kamishak River is in a canyon that drains off the Alaska Peninsula in a south-east direction emptying into the Shelikof Strait across from Kodiak Island. This is an extremely remote river, very difficult to get to and is visited by few people. The only way to really get there is to fly with an experienced and I mean very experienced bush pilot who has flown on the Alaska Peninsula through the Katmai Park. On my three trips to the Kamishak River on three different occasions the trips all started at the Rainbow Lodge on the Kvichak River. It was always a hit or miss proposition as to whether or not you could get into the Kamishak because the weather on the Alaska Peninsula was always unpredictable and could change by the hour. You had to fly south from the Kvichak River over the top of the Alaska Peninsula and head down the canyon where the Kamishak flowed into the Shelikof Strait and then land the float plane in the fairly small pool of water that accumulated at the river's outlet before it flowed across the sandbars into the strait.

You had to return by the same route and make sure that you could get back up the canyon and over the top of the Alaska range ridge into the Kvichak River. That is why an experienced pilot is a must. There were two trips that we could not get into the Kamishak because of the weather, the ceilings being too low to get over the top of the Alaska Peninsula.

The Kamishak River is in the next canyon to the west of the MacNeil River. The MacNeil River has an international reputation as a gathering place for giant Alaskan brown bears. However, at the MacNeil River you have to put in an application and your name has to be drawn from a lottery to be allowed to even go there. Some people wait years before they are selected in the lottery to be able to go into the MacNeil River and then are only allowed only one or two nights at the river and the experience of viewing bears is going to depend a lot on the weather. There are no accommodations there. You have to sleep in a tent. The other famous bear viewing place in the Katmai National Park and Preserve is the Brooks River which has a worldwide reputation for bear viewing and attracts people from all over the world that come there to stay at the Brooks Lodge and view Alaska brown bears from a viewing platform. My wife and I took advantage of this trip one year. When we landed at the Brooks River we had to go through "Bear School" and we learned all the do's and don'ts about being in an area packed with the Alaska brown bear or grizzly who come there during the salmon runs to feast on the fresh fish.

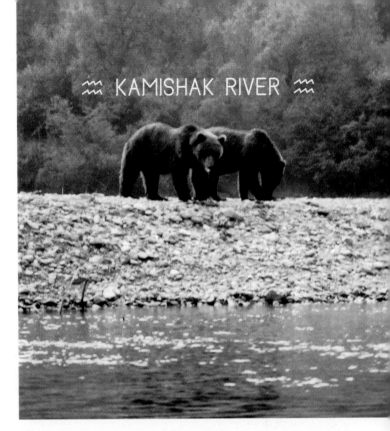

≈ KAMISHAK RIVER ≈

The Kamishak is completely different from the Brooks River and the MacNeil River in its wildness, remoteness and the extreme difficulty in getting there. On our trips once we got over the Alaska Peninsula down the canyon and landed at the a small pool at the outlet of the river we used flat bottom aluminum boats with a 25 horse power engine to travel up the river canyon. The river winds and bends making visibility poor and one can suddenly encounter industrial-size Alaskan brown bears fasting on the salmon particularly in the summer and fall. In addition to the silver salmon run the river is full of large Dolly Varden with beautiful silver sleek bodies and bright pink spots. Earlier in the season there is a pink salmon run so the river is full of giant Alaska brown bear or grizzlies from early summer into the fall. The fishing for both bears and humans is fantastic.

Seeing the large brown grizzly bears there was quite magical as you realize that they are the dominant species in the area. Most of the bears that I saw were very large and very dark and not the least bit intimidated by humans and paid little attention to the humans entering their preserve. The bears came and went as they pleased and were not deterred by our presence. The river itself is not that deep and the bears were not that far away and I felt that if a bear wanted to charge our boat it would have been easy for them with their immense size. If I could visit any of Alaska's wild rivers again the Kamishak would be my first choice as I really relished the opportunity to experience the giant Alaska grizzly in its own element as the grizzly is the epitome of wild Alaska.

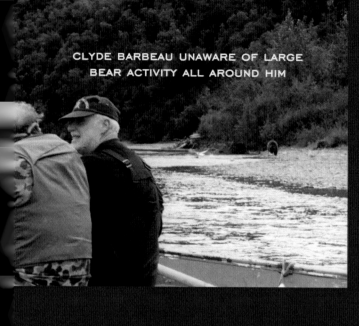

CLYDE BARBEAU UNAWARE OF LARGE
BEAR ACTIVITY ALL AROUND HIM

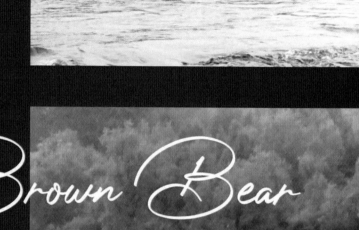

Alaska Brown Bear

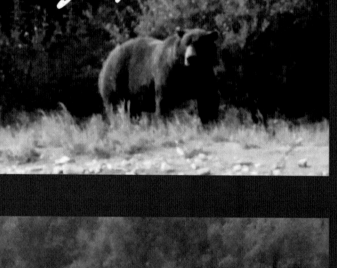

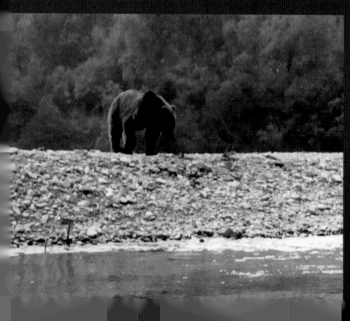

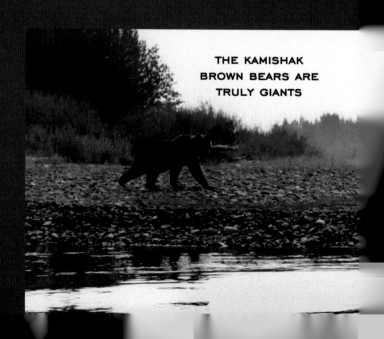

THE KAMISHAK
BROWN BEARS ARE
TRULY GIANTS

As I indicated at the outset of this chapter to really see wilderness Alaska one had to experience the wild scenic untouched rivers of Alaska. Negotiating the rivers of Alaska requires one to leave their comfortable lodges and live in simple tents, sleep on rocky hard ground, endure hardships, face hoards of mosquitoes and other extraordinary risks from being in the wilderness. The persistent challenge of flowing water attracts the adventurous traveler. As I described in my early chapters as a little boy I spent hours on the banks of Kern River daydreaming about what it would be like to travel on the waters of a river. While many rivers do have trails along their banks there are few in Alaska that do. Sometimes the only evidence of people passing on a river is a partially burnt old log or a few black campfire rocks to show someone had been there before. Often there is nothing but the water and the shore and the water leaves no tracks. There is the solitude of the rushing water, sometimes a cloud burst, sometimes a howl of a wolf and at other times the enchanting call of a loon - the permanent recollections that one takes away from these experiences. The Alaska wild really means a sense of being untamed, unadulterated - a place where nature and animals are in balance, where man is a visitor and intruder. All of the rivers that I have navigated are wild in this sense and this is their great attraction and creates their great challenges. The unknown about Alaska rivers is that conditions can change daily often by the hour and what was once a placid river can turn into a hellish nightmare of flowing swift water in a cloud burst of rain. I feel quite blessed to have floated, canoed or kayaked some of the most incredible water ways in wilderness Alaska:

STIKINE RIVER

NOATAK RIVER

BIG MULCHATNA RIVER

LITTLE MULCHATNA RIVER

CHILIKANDRONTNA RIVER

KVICHAK RIVER

WILD RIVER

LAKE CREEK

ALAGNAK RIVER

NUSHAGAK RIVER

NAKNEK RIVER

KOYUKUK RIVER

SAGAVANIRKTOK RIVER

UGASHIK RIVER

KENAI RIVER

KAMISHAK RIVER

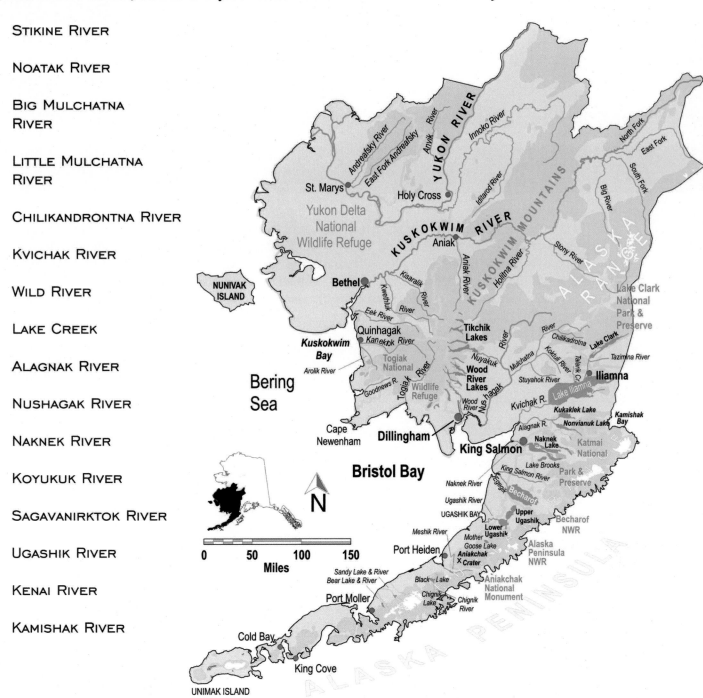

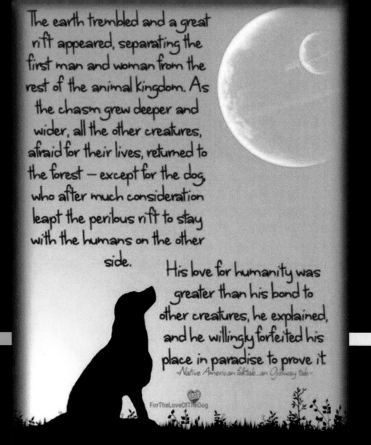

The earth trembled and a great rift appeared, separating the first man and woman from the rest of the animal kingdom. As the chasm grew deeper and wider, all the other creatures, afraid for their lives, returned to the forest — except for the dog, who after much consideration leapt the perilous rift to stay with the humans on the other side.

His love for humanity was greater than his bond to other creatures, he explained, and he willingly forfeited his place in paradise to prove it

~Native American folktale...an Ojibway tale~

ForTheLoveOfTheDog

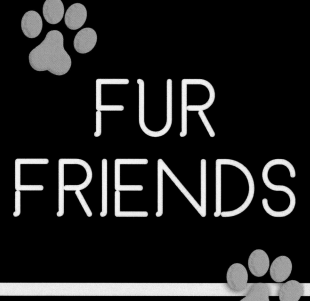

FUR FRIENDS

*O*f the various fur people who have left the great rift to stay with humans on this side I have been fortunate to meet up with and bond with some of the very best. My father bought me a dog on my birthday in May of 1937, a black cocker spaniel named Topper, named after a 1937 movie staring Leo G. Carroll. Topper and I bonded immediately and I would often curl up with him for naps. My parents often remarked that Topper was extremely protective of me as a child and after I learned to walk would shadow me around the house and Lemucchi's Grocery where I would be with my father.

Because of Topper I developed a lifelong love affair for cocker spaniels - my favorite breed of fur people. I don't think there was any other animal as sensitive to human emotions than a cocker. With their long ears and big black emotional eyes they will win your heart in a second. Nonjudgmental, affectionate and beyond loyal they provide a deep unconditional love to their human counterpart.

When Topper left the earth after a long loving relationship he was replaced by a female puppy, a cocker spaniel named Topsy, as cute and as affectionate a little cocker female as you could find. She lived with us for several years but unfortunately passed from an un-treatable doggie illness.

In 1942, our family had moved from behind the Lemucchi's Grocery Store at 725 East 19th Street to a new home in La Cresta with a good size yard and we had Lucky, a male blond and brown cocker, come to live with us. Tonia, my sister, and I loved Lucky and raised him for several years. Unfortunately Lucky was struck by a car and left my sister and me with broken hearts.

Our next dog was not a cocker spaniel but a stray mixed breed who came off the streets and adopted us and became one of the best dogs we ever owned. Tippy, named for the white tip at the end of her tail, was a great family pet, intensely loyal, affectionate and gentle. At the time Tippy came to live with us I was in the seventh grade at Garces Junior High School being taught by the Christian brothers. Tippy would walk the two or three miles from my home to Garces Junior High School and spend the day with me in the classroom. Tippy was quiet and slept under my desk and the Christian brother teachers didn't seem to mind a bit. Occasionally when I was sick and could not go to school Tippy would go in my place and my classmates would let me know that Tippy was at school even though I wasn't there. Tippy was a great companion and stayed with us all through my high school days.

Unfortunately, when I left high school and moved to Palo Alto to attend Stanford University, Tippy could not come and remained home with my mom and dad and sister Tonia. While at Stanford and Georgetown Law School I was not able to have any dogs.

After my wife Margaret and I married in July of 1970 my daughter Lisa came to live with us and I thought it was time to have fur people back in our lives with us again. Our first dog in our new house was a white cocker spaniel named Honey who was an affectionate creature. We also raised rabbits at that time and the rabbits and Honey became good friends.

After Honey came a long line of successful, beautiful cocker spaniels beginning with Penny. Penny was the grand dame of our soon-to-be cocker dynasty. Margaret found Penny when a family in our neighborhood got word out that they had cocker puppies for adoption. We picked out a puppy and named her Penny because of the color of her coat. She was a great family dog, loved our yard and was especially fond of traveling to Mammoth where we had a condominium in the 1970s and to play and roll in the snow in the winter and to swim in the lakes and streams in the summer.

Since my daughter Lisa was living with us we thought it would be fun to have puppies and advertised for a mate for Penny. We heard back from a family that had a male cocker, Beau-Beau XVII, who was a pedigree show dog. We weren't looking for such a fancy mate but agreed with the cocker family that they could have one of the puppies. So in 1974 Penny delivered six puppies for us one of which we gave to Beau-Beau, the sire's family. The whelp or puppy that we kept from the litter we named Peaches. Penny, the mother, and Peaches, the daughter, became lifelong friends both living with us to age sixteen. They were both a delight, enjoyed our home and our swimming pool and our trips to Mammoth. My wife, Margaret, and daughter, Lisa, and I took Penny and Peaches by motor home with us to Alaska where we rafted the Stikine River from Telegraph, British Columbia to Wrangell, Alaska. We borrowed my secretary's motor home and drove up the west coast through California, Oregon and into Washington and caught the inland passage ferry from Seattle to Wrangell, Alaska. In Wrangell we left the two dogs at Mrs. Webb's kennel and did our trip on the Stikine River. Unfortunately the dogs got infested with ticks at the kennel and it was a hassle getting rid of them when we returned to Bakersfield. The trip with the dogs in the motor home was a blast. The dogs stayed in the motor home below the decks on the ferry and twice each day I would go down, put them on their leashes and walk them around the lower decks for them to do their business along with other dog families on the same boat. They adapted to ferry

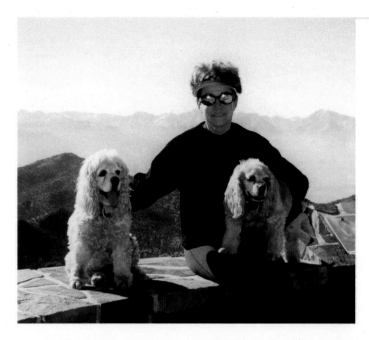

life quite readily and loved Alaska once they got out of the kennel. They were both excellent travel companions. After Penny and Peaches went to dog heaven we felt that we needed to continue to have cocker spaniels and Margaret found Blondie, a puppy that she purchased out of the back of a station wagon that was full of cockers on their way to a dog sale in Los Angeles. Blondie turned out to be a fantastic dog and was quite an athlete. During the time that Blondie was our fur companion I was training for many triathlons and used to run on a regular basis at 6:00 am. I would set the alarm for 5:30 am, roll out of bed, drive out to Lake Ming and do a four to six mile run beginning at 6:00 am, with Blondie right by my side. Blondie got so used to the daily run that she would wake me up by jumping on my bed and licking my face before the alarm would even go off. Blondie was quite a winter dog also and would take ski trips with me to Rock Creek cabin. She also loved cross country skiing at the Obsidian Dome trails between Mammoth and June Lake.

During Blondie's lifetime we had a stray cocker spaniel come into our life that we named Blossom. Blossom was a Shafter stray dog who had wondered into the yard of Margaret's parents' neighbors and seemed to want to stay. The neighbor told Margaret's mother about the dog and said that Margaret loved cocker spaniels and she should call Margaret to see whether Margaret was interested. Of course Margaret was interested and we had Blossom come to live with us. Blondie fortunately accepted Blossom and the two became great friends. Blondie and Blossom probably hiked as many trails and put in as much mileage as any person in the eastern Sierra wilderness. During that time Margaret and I were avid hikers and would often take Blondie and Blossom on five to ten mile hikes with us to an array of beautiful lakes and locations in the eastern Sierra Nevada Mountains.

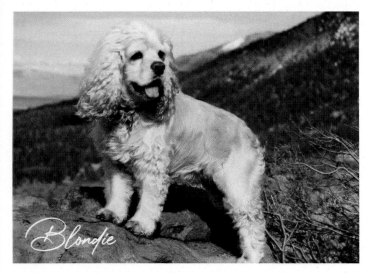

Blondie

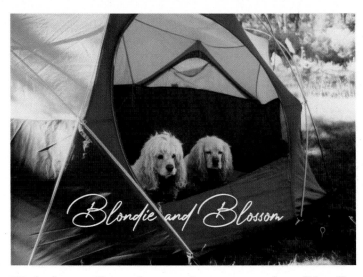

Blondie and Blossom

Blondie and Blossom also loved Rock Creek cabin and I spent many "two dog nights" sleeping on a mat on the floor with my two fur friends. Both Blondie and Blossom lived long wonderful dog lives and left us at age fourteen and fifteen.

Blondie as indicated was quite the runner and became well-trained on her daily runs with me. Blondie and I entered a five mile race at Hart Park which Blondie actually won coming in first at 35 minutes with me holding on to her leash a couple of feet back coming in at second place both having finished in approximately 35 minutes running 7 minute miles.

We had great fun at the award ceremony where Blondie was announced as the winner and received high praise and applause from the crowd as well as a 1st place medal. I receivd the 2nd place medal.

After Blondie and Blossom left us, Margaret and I thought that we really didn't want anymore dogs but as the days passed we both missed the companionship of our fur friends. Margaret saw an ad in the paper that a local woman had some six week old cocker baby puppies for sale. Margaret called me on her way to Los Angeles, told me about the woman and gave me her address, said to go by and look at the puppies and if I thought one of them looked good have the woman reserve the puppy and we would pick the puppy up the following Monday. I went to the woman's home on a Friday morning and visited the puppies which she brought into her den. There were five of them, all little blond cuties - four females and one male. Although Margaret gave me certain instructions I picked one who was the exact image of Blondie and a second who was the exact image of her dam, or her mother. I paid the women for the two dogs and took them home. Margaret reminded me I was only supposed to reserve one dog for approval.

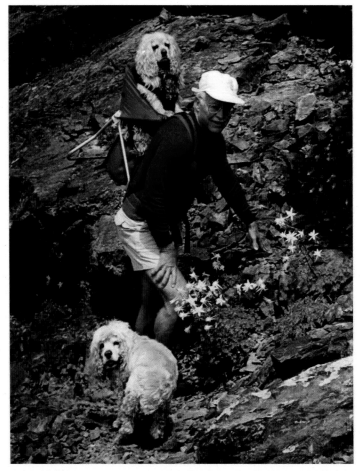

BLOSSOM RECOVERING FROM BACK SURGERY IN THE BACK PACK ON A SIERRA HIKE. BLONDIE BELOW.

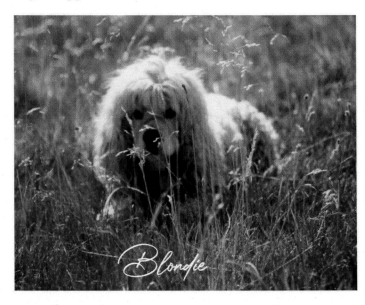

Blondie

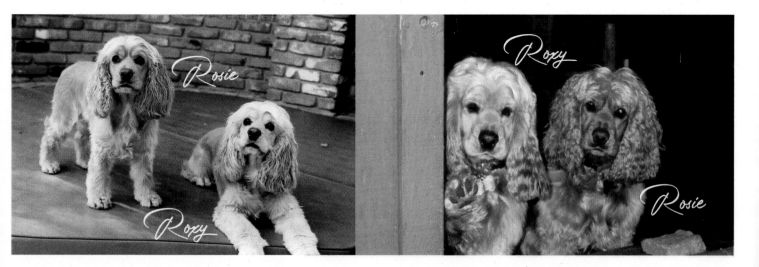

My response to Margaret was that I should have bought all five home! In retrospect I should have.

Even though they were little puppies we took them to Mammoth that weekend to introduce them to the high Sierras. We put them in the bathroom since they were not housebroken and put a fence up in front of the bathroom door. It wasn't long before they learned how to jump up on the fence and knock it down and come running into the room with us to bond with their new human mates. We named the blonde puppy Roxy and the reddish brown puppy Rosie. These two dogs won our hearts immediately and we all became fast friends. They loved hiking, cross country skiing and swimming and particularly being with mommy and daddy. Roxy and Rosie were with us when we moved into our river home and really loved the huge 2.5 acre yard where they could run and play and chase squirrels, racoons and rabbits with abandon. We had a game at our Mammoth Mountain home called bathroom Olympics - the winner was the puppy that could unroll a roll of toilet paper the fastest or pull the most Kleenex from the box the fastest. Both dogs were excellent competitors.

During the last years of Roxy and Rosie's life we were adopted by a stray dog that someone apparently had abandoned on Round Mountain Road near our home. The stray dog was very suspicious and apprehensive about humans approaching her. She would bark and snarl if you got too close. She would sleep in my compost pit outside our fence because it was probably warm there and then come around to check us out suspiciously to determine whether we meant her any harm. Margaret noted that the dog was pregnant, felt sorry for her and began leaving food out for her which she eagerly consumed. That caused the dog to become less apprehensive and come closer although she didn't want anyone touching her or petting her. The dog was a Jack Russell mixed breed white with brown spots on the face-and of course soon became more friendly. I hadn't seen her for several days and I was walking

past my shed in the back of the yard when I heard some squeaks. I investigated and found the noise was coming from under the shed but could not see what was going on. I got a flashlight and saw some little eyes lighting up under the shed in the back corner which only had several inches of clearance. I thought it might be racoon babies or maybe possums or some other creatures. I couldn't reach back far enough so got a long pole and made a loop at the end and lassoed the little creatures which of course turned out to be the puppies of Lulu, our new dog.

I was able to pull out three puppies and called Margaret and told her she was a grandmother. I went back and looked under the shed again and saw more eyes and was able to pull out two more. So there were five in all. We moved Lulu and her puppies up to the back patio and they became an instant attraction for all the neighborhood kids. We were able to find good homes for all of the puppies. Each puppy looked like one of the neighbor's dogs down the road - 1, a golden retriever; 2, a rottweiler; 3, a Labrador; and others a Chihuahua. It appeared that Lulu had many male friends up and down the neighborhood.

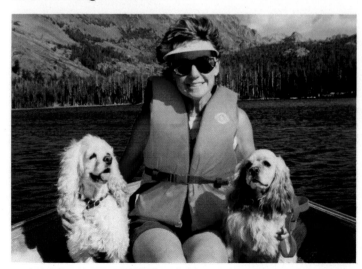

MARGARET AT LAKE MARY, MAMMOTH
WITH BLONDIE AND BLOSSOM

123

Lulu turned out to be a wonderful, affectionate, playful, energetic, loyal dog who stayed with is for many years. Lulu took right up with the program of hiking, cross country skiing and spending time at Rock Creek cabin.

After Roxy passed on Rosie remained but was hampered by old age and arthritis. Lulu became a good companion for the aging Rosie.

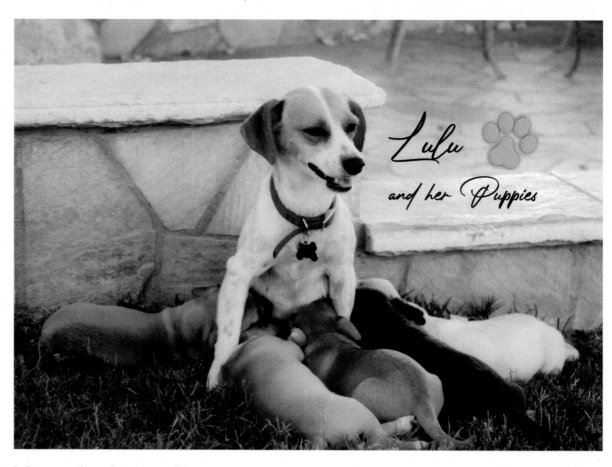

Lulu and her Puppies

After Rosie and Lulu left us we thought we would never have another dog as we were aging and didn't think we wanted to care for a dog especially since we wanted to be away from home occasionally. Well that attitude did not last long and before long Margaret said she saw a dog at the County Animal Shelter that looked promising. She sent me on an errand to check out the dog and told me to reserve it if it looked promising. Well at the shelter I immediately spotted a different dog, a small white Chihuahua that had big black eyes that said: "take me, take me.' I was an easy pushover and made immediate arraignments to take new dog "Susie" to her new, forever home. Susie has turned out to be a real cutie, a playful, fun, affectionate, intelligent, loving little dog and a great choice for our family. After bringing Susie home she had to work out a relationship with Pumpkin, our orange cat, but after awhile that was accomplished. Both have become good friends. Susie is a great walking dog and has given me a new level of regular 1 to 2 hour walks.

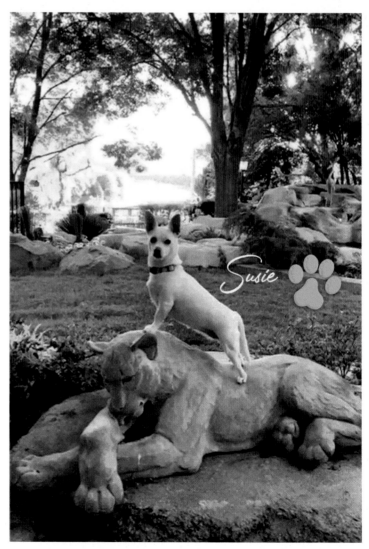

Susie

Our fur friends over the last seventy plus years have given our family close and unconditional bonding and affection. It is so true that these little creatures' love has added immeasurably to a fulfilled life. I look back at running over mountain trails, around lakes, through shady forests and across creeks and skiing ski trails with...my little fur friends as some of the most pleasurable moments of life.

They truly give one a lifetime of joy but do break your heart when they leave us.

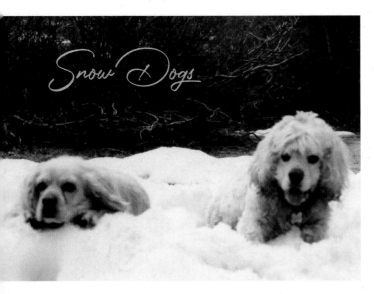
Snow Dogs

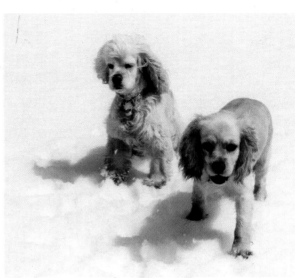

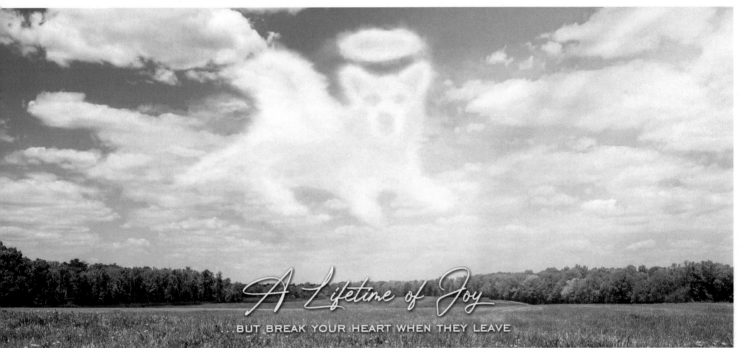
A Lifetime of Joy
...BUT BREAK YOUR HEART WHEN THEY LEAVE

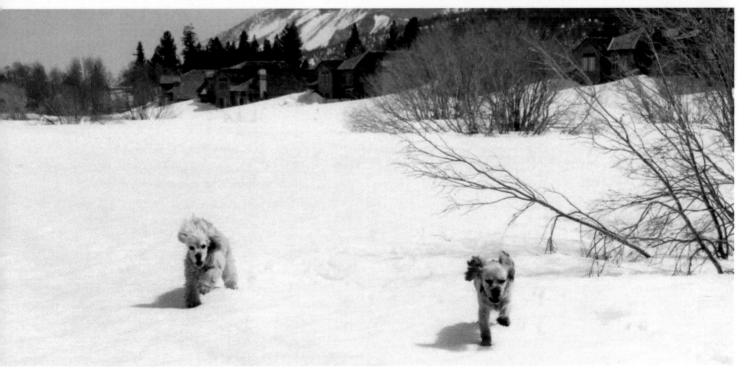

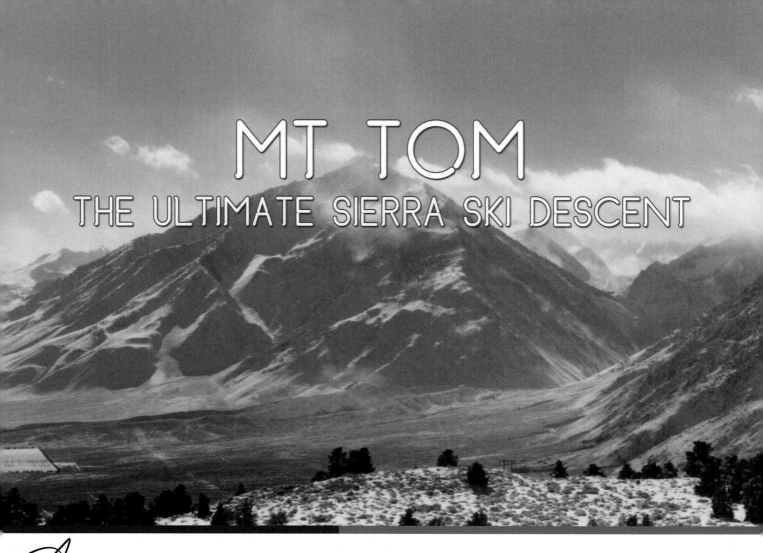

MT TOM
THE ULTIMATE SIERRA SKI DESCENT

*A*nyone who drives south from the Mammoth Lakes junction down US 395 over Sherwin Pass toward Bishop is confronted by the massive mountain Mt. Tom to the west. Rising vertically out of Round Valley to 13,650 feet in one vertical mass it is one of the most impressive mountains on the east Sierra escarpment. In studying the eastern face of Mt. Tom one can see the sweeping "Z" shaped line of Elderberry Canyon leading from just below the summit to the flat plain of Round Valley.

Many of the Sierra backcountry expert skiers call Mt. Tom and Elderberry Canyon the finest peak descent in the Sierra Nevada mountains with a vertical drop of approximately 7,000 uninterrupted feet.

On Easter Sunday, April 6, 1980 I skied Mt. Tom's Elderberry Canyon with my ski mountaineering buddy Doug Robinson.

What made this ski descent so memorable is that Doug and I climbed to the shoulder of the summit of Mt. Tom at approximately 13,000 feet on Nordic "skinny skis" with skins attached to the bottoms. Doug descended the mountain on the same skis without skins, of course. I, however, carried alpine downhill ski boots in my backpack and had strapped to my backpack a pair of Rossignol downhill alpine skis all freshly waxed.

Climbing skins are long pieces of material that are cut to the length of the ski and can either cover the entire bottom or maybe just one or two inches. The skins are then strapped or glued to the bottom of Nordic skis and allow a skier to walk uphill in the snow. The original skins were made of seal fur (hence the name skins). Most modern climbing skins use dense angled synthetic fibers that allow a ski to glide forward but do not allow it to slip backward.

The night before our adventure I spent the night at Doug Robinson's house on Ocean View Avenue near the small mining town of Rovanna in Round Valley just north of Bishop. By 3:00 a.m. Doug and I were out the door in his battered red Volkswagen driving away from Rovanna up the Pine Creek Road in the dark where we exited on a rough dirt road that took us to the base of Elderberry Canyon at about 6,000 feet. At 4:00 a.m. still in the dark we parked off the dirt road and used our Nordic cross-country boots to hike up the ravine toward Elderberry Canyon on a dirt trail. When we reached snow level at about 6,500 feet we put skins on the bottom of our Nordic skis and started our climb on the snow toward the summit of Mt. Tom in the dark. Since Doug had skied Mt. Tom before, he knew the way and guided us along the snow-filled ravine exiting Elderberry Canyon with his headlight. By around 5:30 a.m. we were well into Elderberry Canyon with enough light to pick our way up the bottom of the canyon.

This had been a big snow year in the Sierras. There was good snow coverage, and we plodded up the canyon bottom without obstacles.

The snow was hard-packed and somewhat icy in the early morning cold at around 25 degrees.

Doug broke trail, and we moved up the canyon bottom on an approximately 30 degree slope at a rapid pace.

Doug and I were able to move expeditiously up the steep slope because we were both in fantastic physical condition. Just the week before we had finished a three-week high Sierra crest tour on Nordic skis from Bishop Pass, just west of Bishop, south down the Sierra crest crossing from east to west into the Sequoia National Park and exiting the mountains at Giant Forest, eighteen days and over one hundred miles across some of the steepest and most rugged passes in the high Sierras. We were both "lean and mean" and could maintain a remarkable pace even at altitude.

The ski up the canyon was accomplished in long layered traverses as opposed to heading straight up. The long turns increased the distance but lessened the steepness, and with our supurb conditioning we could skate through the snow which in the middle of the canyon had now turned to easily glidable corn snow.

At about 3/4ths of the way up the canyon there is an abandoned mine - known as the Lambert mine - at 10,850 feet that lies at the center of a monstrous cirque. This area had been mined extensively for tungsten which is used to harden steal. Tungsten mining operations were ongoing in the next canyon to the north - Pine Creek Canyon.

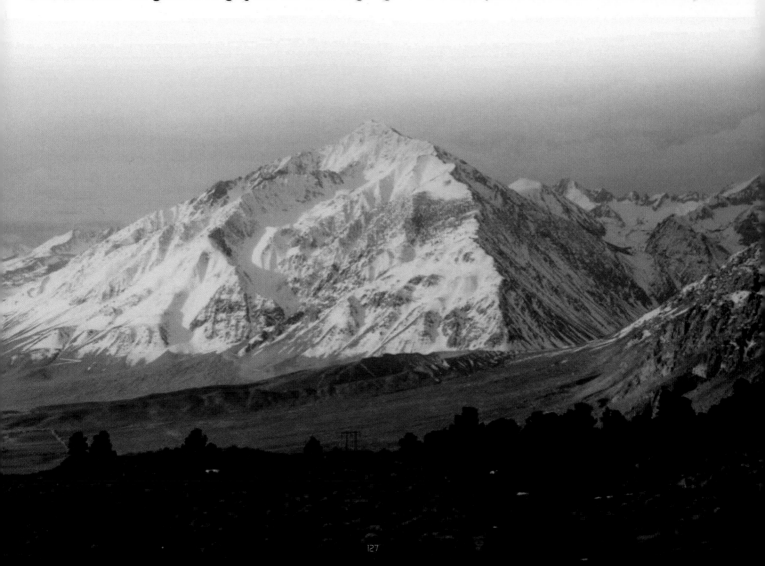

From the mine we climbed up the south-facing side of the cirque which was now very steep and required shorter traverses and changes of lead to break trail in the now-crusted snow.

After some effort we climbed up another 1,000 to 1,200 feet onto the north shoulder of Mt. Tom at about 12,500 feet. We were only a few hundred feet from the summit. It did not look as if we could ski down the north ridge from the top as it was covered in rocky outcrops. We could have climbed to the top without skis.

However, since our goal was really to ski Elderberry Canyon and not go to the summit of Mt. Tom at 13,650 feet we decided to ski off the north shoulder at probably 500 feet from the summit. It was now noon on a crystal clear cold day, Easter Sunday. I dug out a spot in the snow to anchor my rear end and stabilize myself while I changed from my Nordic boots into my alpine downhill ski boots. I re-packed my Nordic boots and put on a light wind proof jacket. I then attached my Rossignol 210 cm skis with alpine bindings and adjusted my ski poles to downhill length. I yelled to Doug, "Let's go!" Doug took off first on his skinny skis, without skins, doing expert telemarks in the hard packed crusty snow. I let Doug get well ahead of me because I knew with my alpine skis pointed downhill and doing parallel turns I could catch him easily.

PHEW! - I inhaled, taking a big gulp of freezing alpine air into my lungs at 13,000 feet. From there on it was an accelerating "e-ticket ride."

With a few long sweeping parallel traverses on hard fast snow I caught up with Doug.

We both screamed with joy.

The beautiful thing about Elderberry Canyon on that day is that the canyon is barrel-shaped, the bottom is flat and there were no obstacles, trees, rock outcrops to interfere with a descent. The depth of the snow was probably 10 to 20 feet in the canyon and covered everything in the bottom of the canyon without any obstacles. Even lower down it must have been in the range of 5 to 10 feet in depth because the snow covered everything including any rock outcrops or bush.

Below the monstrous cirque-which reminded me of the cornice or Scotty's Run at Mammoth Mountain-the snow had turned to corn and was a downhill skier's heaven to glissade on the smooth icy corn with giant parallel turns-kicking up a corn spray behind the ski edges.

Corn snow is large-grained rounded crystals formed from repeated melting and freezing of the snow. On the surface a crust forms that will support one's weight when frozen. I liken it to skiing on thousands of tiny marbles. It is fast but forgiving. The Sierra Nevada at its high altitudes is famous for its spring corn snow - a skier's favorite after powder.

I would stop to catch my breath and watch Doug do his smooth telemarks and parallel turns down the slope kicking up the corn snow. On corn snow, even with Nordic skis and bindings, one can ski parallel turns. A good skier like Doug can do both parallel and telemark.

When we would stop together we would both repeat over and over: "Wow, wow, wow! It doesn't get any better than this."

Unfortunately good things do come to an end. As we skied toward the bottom of the canyon the snow became increasingly softer and thicker so that I now had to fall behind Doug's Nordic tracks that had compressed the snow to keep up any speed.

Toward the end of the canyon we exited on a dirt trail that historically provided access to the Lambert mine. We abandoned our skis, and I switched again to Nordic boots so that I could walk on the dirt trail.

When we got back to the car the day was ended. We loaded up our equipment, popped the lids on two cans of ice cold beer we had stashed for the occasion and began the slow bumpy ride back to Rovanna and civilization.

Having a second home at Mammoth Lakes for many years I am frequently on Highway 395 north and south passing by Mt. Tom. Every time I look at Elderberry Canyon I can visualize that 6,000 foot glissade down through the corn snow. When I have time I like to stop at the overlook on US 395, stare at Elderberry Canyon and relive that memorable downhill run turn by turn through Elderberry Canyon. Yes, I'll add my vote - the greatest ski descent in the Sierras.

Mt. Tom is named for Thomas Clark, a resident of the pioneer town of Owensville, who was credited with being the first to climb the peak in the 1860s. Mt. Tom is in the John Muir wilderness.

Unfortunately on March 26, 2005 five skiers in Elderberry Canyon were caught in two separate avalanches. One skier was injured, and two skiers were buried and killed. It can be a dangerous mountain under certain conditions.

But on Easter Sunday in April 1980 Mt. Tom and Elderberry Canyon were the greatest vertical ski descent in the eastern Sierra Nevadas.

SKIING THE CREST OF THE SIERRAS

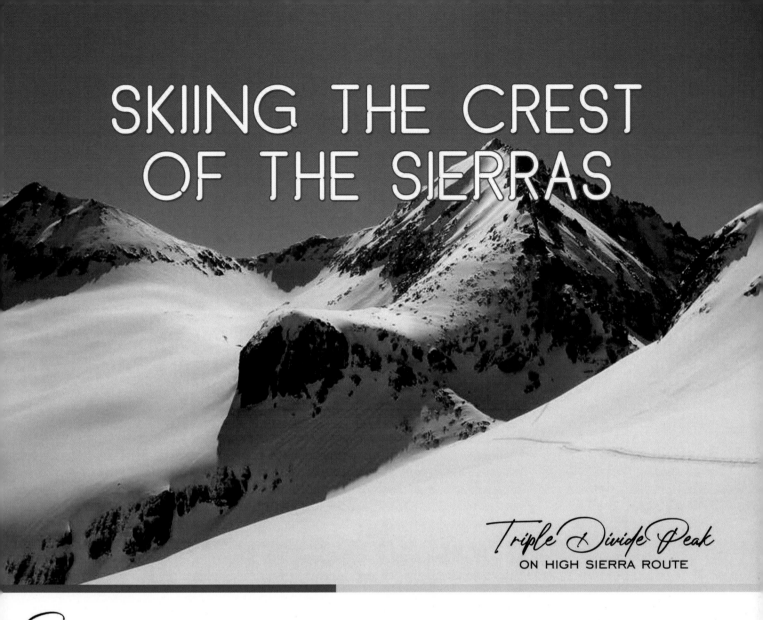

Triple Divide Peak
ON HIGH SIERRA ROUTE

Skiing the crest of California's Sierra Nevada Mountains had been a longtime ambition. Since my first forays into these magnificent mountains as a teenager I had always wondered what it would be like to explore them in the winter months. For most people the winter Sierras are a terra incongnita to be avoided and only entered or crossed in the winter in a warm heated automobile or maybe for the more adventurous the groomed slopes of a ski resort in warm designer clothing with a retreat after a few hours back to a warm lodge and safety.

The high crest of the Sierra Nevadas generally ranges from Mt. Dana in the north at 13,068 feet near the eastern entrance to the Yosemite National Park, south to the Giant Forest in the Sequoia and Kings Canyon National Park. Along the crest of that range are many spectacular peaks including North Palisades at 14, 248 feet; Mt. Humphrey at 13,992 feet; Mt. Williamson at 14,379 feet; Mt. Whitney at 14,500 feet; Mt. Kaweah at 13,807 feet; Mt. Pinchot at 13,500 feet and other spectacular peaks over 10,000 feet.

The Sierra Nevada crest, a magnificent skyline with spectacular landscapes, is one of the most beautiful mountain ranges in the world. The distance from Mt. Dana at the north end of the crest to the Giant Forest at the south end is approximately 200 miles. In the summer these beautiful mountains draw flocks of visitors, hikers and campers to roam the summer trails, lakes, meadows and forests. The mountains are alive with visitors in the summer and fall.

But after the first snowfall in late October or by mid December the summer visitors are gone. In the winter the Sierra Nevada Mountains are a completely different place. From mid November to the snow melt in May, June or July the high Sierras are empty of people except for those with ski mountaineering experience, proper equipment and winter skills. For the ski mountaineers the winter opens up some 200 miles of some of the most spectacular winter mountain environment on the planet, almost completely devoid of people.

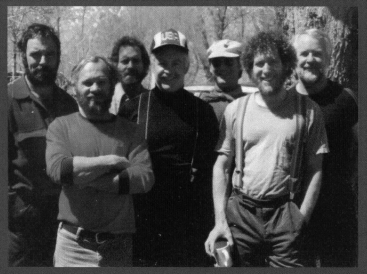

NIGHT BEFORE THE TRIP AT DOUG'S HOME
IN ROUND VALLEY - LEFT TO RIGHT:
JOHN PULSKAMP, DOUG ROBINSON, TIM LEMUCCHI,
AJ MARSDEN, TOM ANDERSON AND KEN JENNINGS

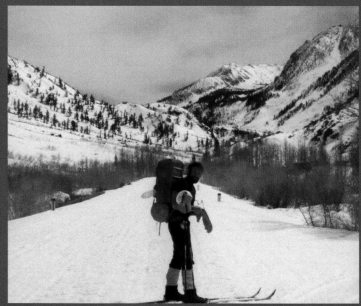

THE BEGINNING OF THE TRIP OF OVER 100 MILES

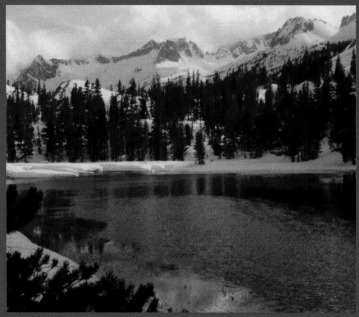

THROUGH THE LAKES BELOW BISHOP PASS

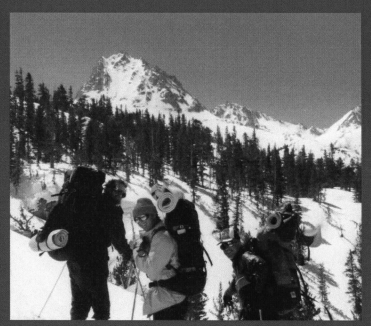

BISHOP PASS AHEAD

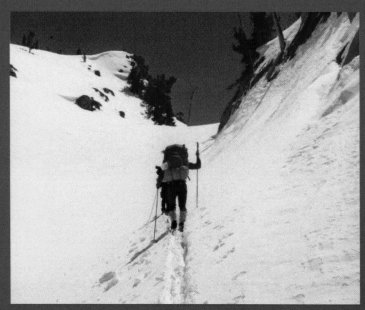

ROUTE OF THE SUMMER TRAIL UP TO THE PASS

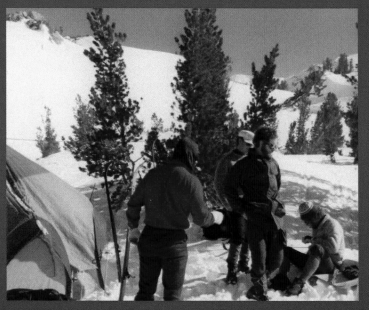

FIRST CAMPSITE

The reason is not complicated. In the winter Sierra Nevada snowfalls are measured in tens of feet. It is fairly common for a single storm to drop 3 to 5 feet of snow, and drops of 10 feet or more are not uncommon. Accumulated snowfall from November to March can reach 10 to 30 feet with record snowfalls in March the rule rather than the exception. Wind gusts over the highest passes often exceed 100 miles per hour. Except for the protected ski areas and their warm lodges the winter Sierras can be a dangerous and hostile place for the untrained, unprepared and inexperienced visitor. But for the hearty few who have ski mountaineering skills, equipment and training, ski tours in the Sierras are a spectacular and memorable experience.

Skiing the crest of the Sierra Nevada Mountains has been a lifelong project for me. As said the distance from Mt. Dana in the north to the Giant Forest on the south along the crest is approximately 200 miles. The distance of the summer John Muir Trail from Yosemite to its end at Mt. Whitney portal is about the same - 211 miles. Needless to say traversing the Sierra crest in the summer season and the winter season are entirely different experiences. In the winter one must know High Sierra weather patterns, avalanche conditions, the best winter skis and camping equipment, how to get to or erect shelter quickly and have the mountaineering skills for a successful back country winter trip experience. Physical strength and conditioning are also necessary for skiing in the back country often in extreme weather conditions.

Accumulating these varied skills took me years to develop and perfect. Thanks largely to my friend Doug Robinson, my years of developing Alpine skiing skills, my years at Rock Creek cabin developing Nordic skiing skills and my training and experience as a triathlete I was able to accomplish the longtime goal of skiing the Sierra crest from Mt. Dana to the Giant Forest. I did not do it all in one excursion but in segments which I describe herein.

My first attempt at a High Sierra ski tour adventure was a failure. This was in 1973 with Doug Robinson and my orthopedic doctor friend Kenneth Jennings. We had the goal of Nordic skiing into Thousand Island Lake on the John Muir Trail at 9,800 feet for a few days of camping and ski touring. We started that venture from the June Lake Loop across from Silverlake at 7,600 feet where we climbed up the Brush Creek Canyon behind the Edison Power Plant. Our equipment in retrospect was pretty primitive: leather boots and 210 cm skis with cable bindings. We simply climbed up the extremely steep side of Brush Creek behind the Edison Power Plant and muscled our way through deep snow to Gem Lake. We skied across the top of frozen Gem Lake and

eventually made our way to the frozen-over Waugh Lake further up the Brush Creek Canyon. Unfortunately it began to snow, and as we forged ahead the snow became thicker and heavier. Skiing in the deepening snow became very difficult so we decided to bivouac for the remainder of the day. After setting up the tent the heavy snow would press the top of the tent down causing dripping water to come into the interior making it wet. We spent a damp and cold night. The next day we attempted some skiing, but the snow was too deep and heavy and we were bogged down. We spent two nights in the tent under extremely cold and windy storm conditions and decided correctly to abort our first attempt to penetrate the High Sierras in the winter.

The next venture was a success. In 1975 Doug Robinson and I planned to ski across the Sierras from Mammoth Mountain to Yosemite. We started our trip at Mammoth Mountain Ski Resort and skied up the Devil's Post Pile Road to the Minaret Vista and then skied north up the San Joaquin Ridge to Deadman's Pass where we headed westbound on the high ridge above the San Joaquin River where we camped for the night. The next day we had excellent snow, deep and well-packed and easily skiable. We skied briskly along the San Joaquin Ridge into the Thousand Island Lake Basin where we spent our second night. The next day from Thousand Island Lake we contoured up to the Donohue Pass on the John Muir Trail and crossed over at 11,000 feet into the Yosemite National Park. From the Donohue Pass we transversed westward onto the Lyell Glacier. We spent the day climbing up the glacier and skiing down its face with some wonderful skiing in well-packed corn snow. We slept that night on the glacier in our sleeping bags on air mats without a tent. The next day we headed down the Lyell Canyon and onto the Lyell fork of the Tuolumne River. The river was frozen over with a few feet of icy snow on top. The ice on the top of the river was strong enough to hold our weight, but it was a somewhat unsettling sensation as we skied down the river channel because you could hear the water running below your skis, particular when we went over falls. You never knew whether you would hit a soft spot and go through the ice into the icy river water below. We were fortunate, however, to stay on the solidly frozen part of the riverbed which supported our weight. The sound of the water running underneath our skis, was a completely surreal event. We camped that night on he snowy banks of the Lyell fork of the Tuolumne River. The next morning we again started down the river channel and skied through a grove of aspens whose leaves and branches were covered in ice. The morning sun from the west caused the ice on the leaves and branches to light up almost as if they were electrified.

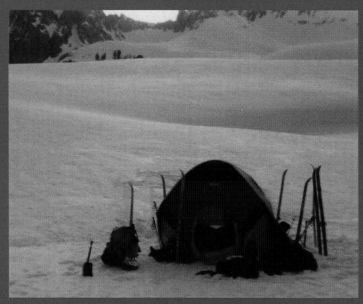

SNOW CAMP

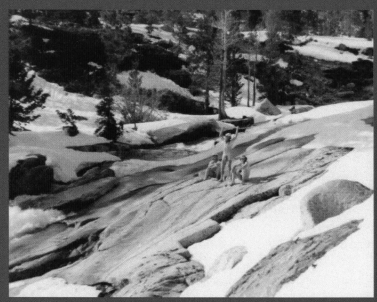

WOOD'S CREEK - OPEN WATER, BATH AND FRESH TROUT

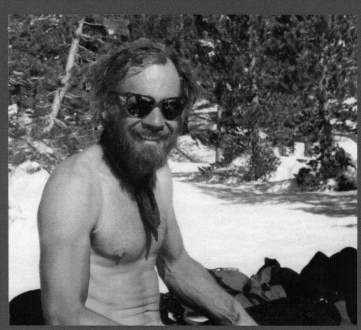

DOUG ROBINSON AFTER BATH IN THE SUNSHINE

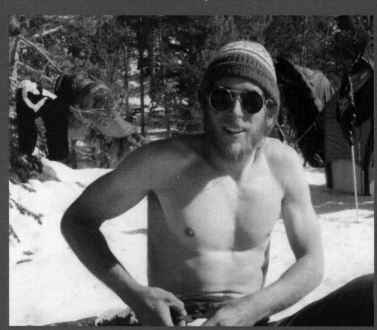

TOM ANDERSON AT WOOD'S CREEK AFTER BATH

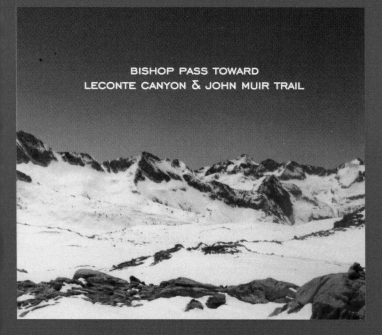

BISHOP PASS TOWARD
LECONTE CANYON & JOHN MUIR TRAIL

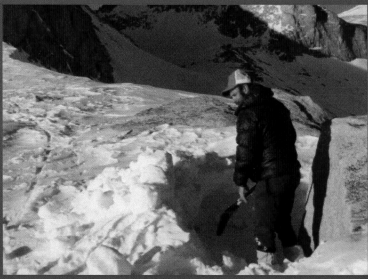

SNOW CAVE WHERE TIM LEMUCCHI AND JOHN PULSKAMP
SPENT THE NIGHT AFTER FIERCE WINDS BLEW TENT
APART ON THIRD NIGHT OUT

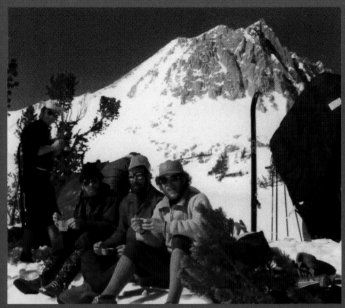

ENJOYING HOT TEA BREAK

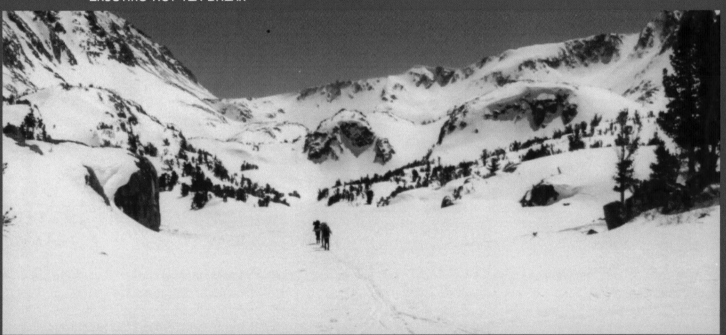

HEADING TOWARD BISHOP PASS.   10,758 FIRST MAJOR PASS.

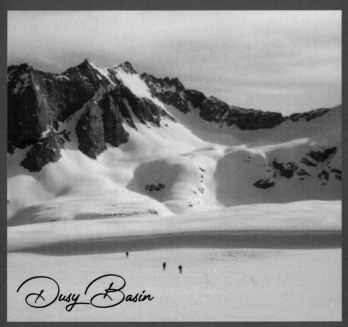

Dusy Basin

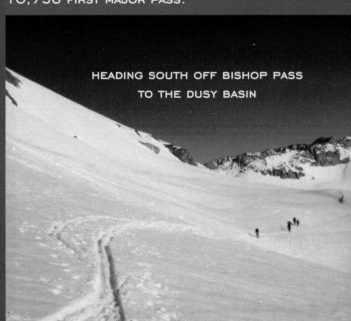

HEADING SOUTH OFF BISHOP PASS
TO THE DUSY BASIN

It was a memorable sight. We eventually reached Tuolumne Meadows and camped at the bridge crossing the Tuolumne River. We then skied down the Yosemite highway covered with 4 to 5 feet of snow toward Tenaya Lake. When we arrived at Tenaya Lake it was getting late in the afternoon and we were hoping to make Yosemite before nightfall. We were five days out of Mammoth, and it was quite windy at the lake. The wind was blowing from east to west quite forcibly. The lake was completely iced over with just a few inches of corn snow on top of the ice which held our weight without any problem. We pulled out a tarp with Doug holding on to one end and me holding onto the other and maneuvered ourselves out into the wind. The wind picked up the tarp like a sail. We kept our skis on and "snow ski sailed" across Tenaya Lake in about thirty-five or forty minutes. What a trip! Had we taken the regular highway route up around the north shore of the lake which was very avalanche-prone it probably would have taken us the rest of the day and evening. Because of our wind-blown excursion across Tenaya Lake we were able to make it down into the Yosemite Valley as it was getting dark and just about cocktail time. After five days on the winter trail we were ready for gin martinis and skied to the Ahwahnee Hotel and saluted our successful trans-Sierra trip by downing several icy cold martinis.

It was pre-planned that my wife Margaret would pick us up in Yosemite. We enjoyed a great meal and a good night sleep at the hotel after a successful crossing of the Sierras.

Being blown across Tenaya Lake was a spectacular and unique experience that I have never forgotten. After that trip Nordic skiing became a favorite sport, and I developed a considerable amount of back country skiing experience and was excelling in the use of newly devel

oped technology in Nordic skis, boots, winter mountaineering and camping equipment.

I completed the northern sections of the Sierra crest on a trans-Sierra tour with Doug Robinson, Tim Anderson and AJ Marsden. We began that trip at Virginia Lakes which is in the last canyon before one crosses Conway Summit on Highway 395 above Mono Lake. We started our trip on the road to Virginia Lakes where we parked at the snow line and climbed from Virginia Lakes at 9,700 feet approximately 6 miles to Summit Pass at 11,000 feet where we camped. The next day we skied into Saddlebag Lake where we skied across the frozen lake and camped at the south end. The next day we skied to the Tioga Pass Road and skied up Highway 120 in deep snow to the entrance to the Yosemite National Park at 9,945 feet where we spent the day skiing the lower slopes of Mt. Dana. We then skied down the Tioga Highway which was covered with 5 to 6 of snow to Tuolumne Meadows. We snow camped there, and the next day skied up the Lyell Fork of the Tuolumne River again camping on the Lyell glacier where we skied the glacier. We then crossed the Sierras at Donohue Pass at 7,056 feet skiing down into Thousand Lakes. From there we traversed across the San Joaquin Ridge and skied down into the Mammoth Mountain Ski Resort.

I completed the central section of the Sierra crest from Mammoth Lakes to Rock Creek Canyon with Doug Robinson. On that trip we skied out of Mammoth Lakes over Duck Pass to Duck Lake then Pika Lake and camped at the top of McGee Creek Canyon. The next day we actually backed down a snow filled chute since it was too steep to ski and got ourselves down into the McGee Creek Canyon. There we skied down the canyon and went south to Steelhead Lake where we crossed over into Pioneer Basin.

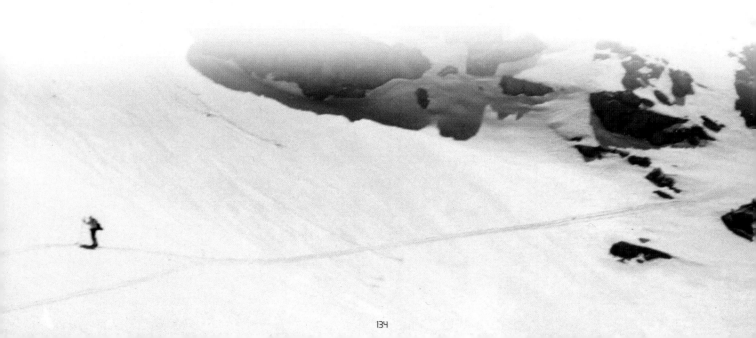

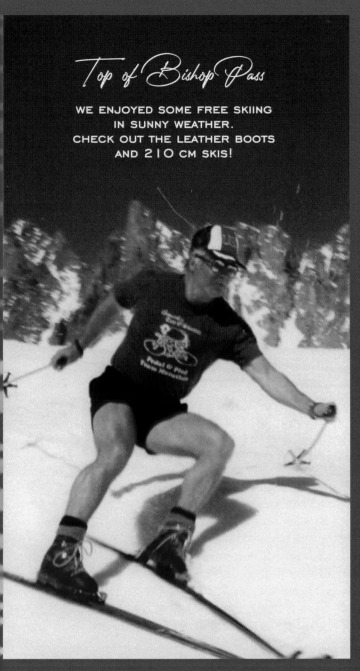

Top of Bishop Pass

WE ENJOYED SOME FREE SKIING
IN SUNNY WEATHER.
CHECK OUT THE LEATHER BOOTS
AND 210 CM SKIS!

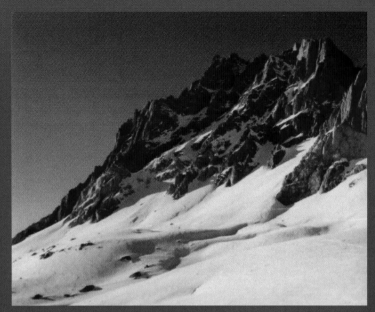

THE WESTSIDE OF THE PALISADES

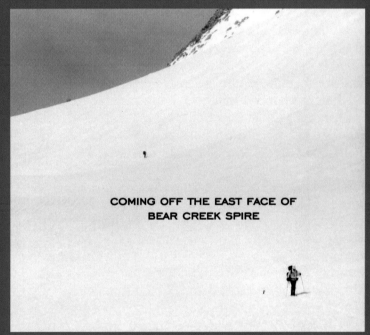

COMING OFF THE EAST FACE OF
BEAR CREEK SPIRE

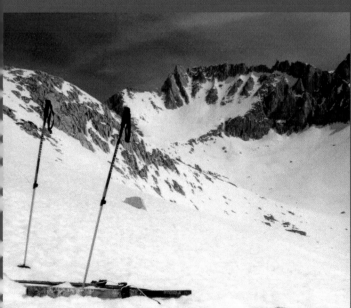

BEAR CREEK SPIRE PASS

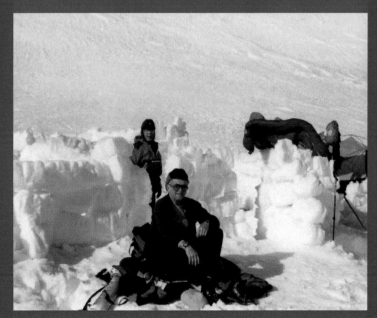

IGLOO CAMP AT LAKE ITALY

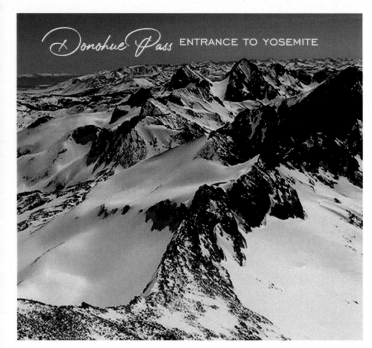

From Pioneer Basin we skied over to Mono Creek and up Mono Creek to Mono Pass at 10,597 feet where we crossed over into Rock Creek Canyon. From Mono Pass we skied down into the Bear Creek Spire cirques and then down the Rock Creek Canyon to the Rock Creek cabin at 10,000 feet.

I completed the mid portion of the Sierra crest from Rock Creek to Bishop Creek with Gary McCain and Don Williams in 1997 on a seven day ski trek from Piute Pass to Rock Creek. We started that trip at North Lake where we were able to drive to the snow line, left our vehicle and then loaded up our 50 pound packs with skis and poles attached and walked as far as we could on the Piute Pass trail before putting on our skis. With skis we followed the route of the summer trail around Mt. Emerson at 13,225 feet tracking up the north fork of Bishop Creek crossing the frozen Loch Laven and Piute Lakes topping out at Piute Pass at 11,000 feet. From the pass we descended down the backside of the flanks of Mt. Humphrey and found a sheltered place to camp. The views of the westside of Mt. Humphrey at 13,992 feet were spectacular especially in the lake afternoon setting sun. We enjoyed a hot dinner and were very tired from the exhausting climb over Piute Pass and all slept soundly.

The next day we had a mellow Nordic ski day skiing across numerous frozen lakes in the Humphrey Basin staying east of Pilot Knob, a peak at 12,245 feet, and camping on the east shore of Alsace Lake. There we built ice block walls to protect our tent from the strong winds. That evening we could see the Pinnacles, a north-south mountain ridge, rising in a stunning formation above Piute Canyon in the late alpenglow.

The next day we skied across the upper or north end of

French Canyon and made the long climb up to Royce Lakes transversing from there over into the Granite Park Basin where we camped.

After a good breakfast and an early morning start we headed up to Italy Pass at 12,400 feet, a real grind. At the top of Italy Pass we skied down the west-facing flanks of the mountain to Jumble Lake and then onto Lake Italy where I had one of the greatest Nordic ski runs ever. The area from Granite Basin to the top of Italy Pass and down to Lake Italy is usually filled with rock slides and large boulders in the summer but in 1977, a heavy snow year, the 45 degree slope from the top of Italy Pass to Jumbo Lake and down to Lake Italy was covered with 10-20 feet of packed snow and on this day all the boulders, rocks and trees were buried. The top surface of the packed snow, however, when we topped over the 12,400 foot Italy Pass, was covered with delightful corn snow and I glissaded down the 50 degree pitch slope in long Nordic parallel and tele-marks turns without any obstacles all the way to Lake Italy. What an incredible run! If only the high Sierras had chairlifts I would have definitely taken a second run. Lake Italy was named because its shape is similar to that of the Italian peninsula, like a boot. At Lake Italy we again built igloo shelters to protect from the constant winds. The next day we intended to make Rock Creek Cabin but inadvertently skied up the wrong canyon and found ourselves in the First Recess headed toward Mono Creek. By the time we realized our error and reversed our course we had lost a great deal of the day. It was becoming increasingly cold and windy as we climbed up the backside of the Bear Creek Spire at 13,700 feet. At the top of the Spire we were dismayed to find the eastside of the Spire almost a vertical wall and too steep to ski down.

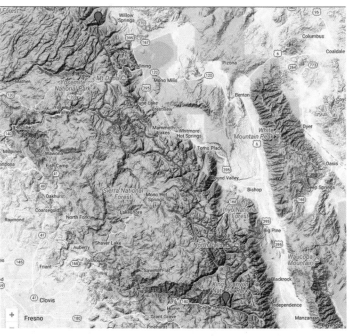

ROUTE OF THE HIGH SIERRA CREST

It would have been miserable to spend the night at the top of Bear Creek Spire Pass at 13,000 feet in frigid cold and wind. I borrowed the maneuver I learned from Doug Robinson on the McGee Creek Canyon. I took off my skis, put my poles in my pack, got some rope and had Gary McCain let out the rope for me as I backed down the slope one step at a time putting both skis deep into the snow, holding onto the skis and rope and then letting one leg down as far as I could, kicking a toe-hold in the face of the wall, making sure it would hold me then pulling up the skis and driving them again deep into the snow below me as far as I could reach then holding onto the skis and repeating the same maneuver with the other foot making steps as far down as the rope would let me. When I had gotten to the end McCain pulled up the rope and it was McCain and Williams' turn to follow me down the holes that I had kicked in the side of the slope. Later on both McCain and Williams told me that the first 50 feet down the slope was terrifying. When I eventually kicked my way down the slope to where it was skiable I stomped out a platform, put on my skis and headed toward more skiable terrain. McCain and Williams followed and we all made it safely down the canyon to where we could camp for one more night. I was asked whether I was sure that as I backed down the slope and kicked foot holes that the snow face would not give way and cause me and perhaps an avalanche to cascade us all in a heap to the bottom of the slope. My answer, " I wasn't sure." The next day we were able to complete the trip. That venture completed the mid portion of the Sierra crest.

Doug Robinson was putting together a trip to ski the southern end of the Sierra crest in April of 1980 and I of course joined up. The starting group included Doug Robinson, Tom Allen, AJ Marsden, John Pulskamp, M.D. and Ken Jennings, M.D. We all started the trip together on April 18, 1980, but not all of us finished at Giant Forrest in Sequoia National Park. The trip began with a rousing farewell party at Doug Robinson's home in Round Valley. The next morning we were driven to the Bishop Creek area and took the South Lake Road as far as we could drive until the road was blocked with snow. We started our trip at the snow line on the road to South Lake. The first part of the trip was getting used to our skis and equipment, making sure all of our packs were securely positioned and packed and acclimating ourselves to the increasing elevation.

When I look back at the photographs we took of that trip I am astonished by the equipment that we used. I was wearing heavy leather boots and using Hexcel 210 cm skis with cable bindings. No one uses leather boots any more, and no one uses 210 cm skis.

We all looked like something out of old ski history books with our equipment. The equipment was heavy and clumsy. The boots and skis nowadays are so much superior in design, weight and utility. It is amazing looking back how we could climb some of the passes and particularity ski down the steep backsides of the passes with the equipment we were using. We made up for the poor performing gear by being young and strong and in great physical condition

We headed up the South Lake Road, skied across South Lake which was frozen over and headed up toward Bishop Pass skiing across the series of lakes leading up to Bishop Pass area. The lakes were frozen over with more than five feet of snow on top so we just skied across them up to the end of tree line for our first camp. Doug Robinson had prepared food in advance and we ate quite lavishly the first night. The next day we headed up toward Bishop Pass at 11,972 feet, our first major pass on the trip. At the top of Bishop Pass you could look west toward LeConte Canyon, the route of the John Muir Trail. We spent some time near the top of Bishop Pass doing some freelance skiing in the bowl on the east side of the pass. We left our packs at the bottom of the bowl and climbed to the top of the pass un-weighted and made several runs. The weather was delightful - sunny and warm with cold snow.

As we descended Bishop Pass and skied south toward the Palisades the weather began to deteriorate so we stamped out a camp on the west side of the Palisades Mountains. That night a major storm struck and blew one of our tents apart.

We all jammed into one tent and slept uncomfortably on top of one another. We buried the remains of the damaged tent the next morning and continued south along the backside of the Palisades where we established our third camp. The storm was still brewing with strong winds and snow. Since we were down to one tent John Pulskamp and I dug a snow cave and spent the night in the cave. The wind blew quite forcefully that night and blew a fine "snow dust" into the cave which penetrated the zipper of my sleeping bag. I spent most of the night scooping up the fine snow off my chest in my bag, crunching it into a snowball and throwing it out the zipper of my sleeping bag. Not too much sleep that night either - very cold. The next day John Pulskamp and Ken Jennings departed and went back to Bishop Pass to return to Bakersfield since they had not "signed-up" for the entire trip.

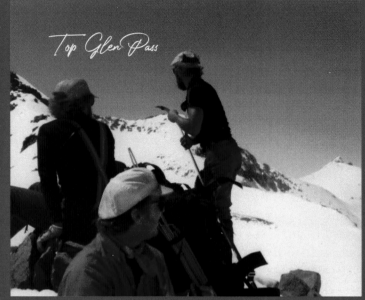

Top Glen Pass

ONE OF THE WORST, ICY AND SLIPPERY 11,900 FEET

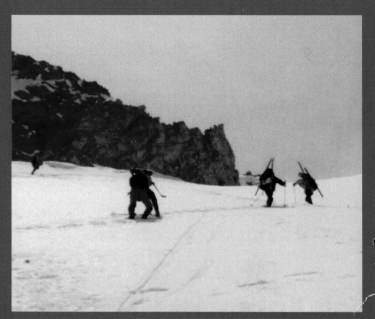

CLIMBING UP MILESTONE BOWL

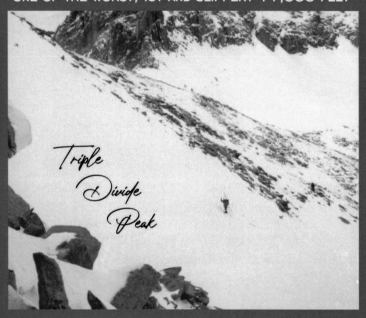

Triple Divide Peak

CIRCUMVENTING TRIPLE DIVIDE PEAK

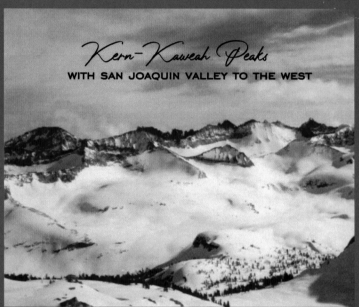

Kern-Kaweah Peaks
WITH SAN JOAQUIN VALLEY TO THE WEST

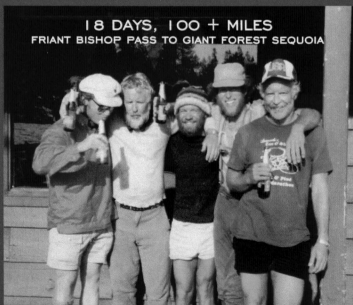

18 DAYS, 100 + MILES
FRIANT BISHOP PASS TO GIANT FOREST SEQUOIA

KEN JENNINGS (NOW DECEASED) AND TIM LEMUCCHI

END OF TRIP APRIL 25, 1980
LEFT TO RIGHT: AJ MARSDEN, KEN JENNINGS,
DOUG ROBINSON, TOM ANDERSON, TIM LEMUCCHI